Anatomy & Physiology for Paramedics

by Stephen Dolphin

illustrated by Valerie Hamilton

Anatomy & Physiology for Paramedics
By Stephen Dolphin
Illustrated by Valerie Hamilton

Second edition
Published by and ©1995
Dolphin Books
South Woodham Ferrers,
Essex, CM3 5TX
Email dolphin@delphis.demon.co.uk

ISBN 0-9520339-0-9

British Library Cataloguing-in-Publication Data
A catalogue record for this book is available from the British Library

Contents

Contents

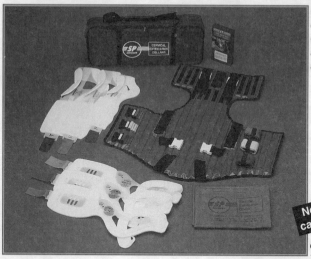

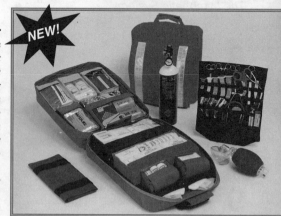

Cells & Tissues

Cell structure

Tissues

Organisation

Basics

The fundamental function of a cell is to take in substances, act upon them or combine them with other substances and then to send the altered or combined substances out into the body.

All living matter is made up of individual cells, the smallest units of life which can function and reproduce themselves. These cells only perform the various essential functions by becoming specialised. Cells have become as diverse as a one metre long neuron and a leucocyte only 8 microns (0.000008 metre) in diameter. They have become dependant on an environment around them which is closely controlled.

All cells have the same basic structure. They are bounded by a thin but very complex semi-permeable cell membrane which selectively controls the entry and exit of thousands of different substances from the cell. These substances pass in and out of the cell by various methods (see later), and act on other substances in the cell to produce the desired new substance. These substances range from a few atoms of a chemical such as potassium or calcium, to complex protein molecules

The interior components (organelles) of the cell are suspended in cytoplasm. This is a thick jelly-like fluid, containing filaments and particles which make up a matrix that physically supports and aids the movement of the organelles. The cytoplasm is also the medium for many chemical reactions within the cell. It is made up of 90% water, (intracellular water accounts for 45% of body weight), with dissolved amino acids, carbohydrates and peptides. Colloids, which will not dissolve in water, are suspended in the fluid, kept separate by their opposing electrical charges.

Cell Components

The cell contains many organelles, or structures, that perform very specific functions. The diagram shows only one or two of each of the main types, but cells contain hundreds or sometimes thousands of organelles, the number and type depending on the type and position of the cell.

Cytoplasm

Cytoplasm is a highly complex substance. It is a thick, jelly-like substance which has an integral framework of very large protein molecules, in the form of filaments and particles, in which lipids and carbohydrates are included. The main bulk of the material is a dilute solution of electrolytes, which are divided into cations and anions. The principal cation (positively charged ion) in the intracellular fluid is potassium (K^+). The principal anions (negatively charged ions) are Chloride (Cl^-), Bicarbonate (HCO_3^-) and Hydroxyl (OH^-). Cytoplasm is the medium for many of the chemical reactions that take place in the cell, which alter substances before they reach the organelles. The actual chemical composition of the cytoplasm is adjusted to suit the requirements of the cell and the organism by taking in or giving out ions through the cell membrane.

Nucleus

The nucleus is surrounded by a nuclear membrane, which performs much the same function as the cell membrane. It contains the nucleoplasm, D.N.A. and chromatin, which are participants in cell division and growth. Prior to reproduction chromatin shortens and coils into rod-like bodies called chromosomes.

Mitochondrion

Mitochondria are the "power house" of the cell. They contain enzymes which convert foods, which have been broken down by the digestive system and transported to the cell, into energy-rich compounds. These compounds are then used within the cell or transported around the body for use in other cells. Cells that use a large amount of energy, such as muscle cells, have a large number of mitochondria, whereas (relatively) inactive bone cells have few.

Centrosome

The centrosomes contain centrioles, which participate in cell division (mitosis).

Granules

These give the cell a speckled appearance under the microscope. They are thought to be food particles in storage until required to repair or replace worn out protoplasm, although this is uncertain.

Vacuoles

Vacuoles derive their name from the fact that they are small pockets in the cytoplasm. They may contain waste materials and secretions, which are then transported outside the cell, usually by pinocytosis.

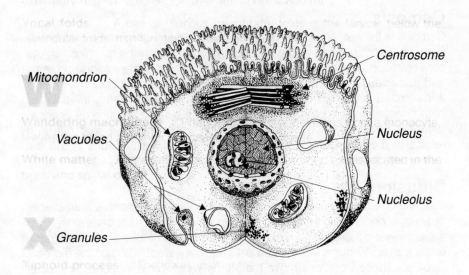

Figure 1-1   A Generalised Cell

Transport across the Cell Membrane

There are several methods of transporting substances across the cell (plasma) membrane, depending on the permeability of the membrane and the size of the molecules or atoms to be transported. The permeability can be adjusted by altering the chemical make-up of the membrane or opening certain channels which will only allow the passage of certain chemicals. Some molecules are soluble in the lipid membrane, whilst some need carriers to take them across.

Passive Processes

Osmosis

Osmosis is the net movement of water across a semi-permeable membrane from an area of low solute concentration to an area of high solute concentration. The water passes through channels in the integral proteins and dissolves through the membrane directly. An important point to note is that osmosis is the NET movement of water. Water is constantly travelling in both directions across the cell membrane for the same reasons as occur in diffusion. The difference between diffusion and osmosis is that diffusion results in the net movement of solutes, whilst osmosis results in the net movement of water.

Diffusion

This is the net movement of solutes across a semi-permeable membrane, down the concentration gradient, from an area of higher concentration to an area of lower concentration. This is achieved by the natural Brownian Motion of the atoms. All atoms vibrate at a set frequency, depending on the element involved. These vibrations move the atoms in random directions. The result of a higher concentration on one side of a semi-permeable membrane is that there are more movements across the membrane towards the area of low concentration simply because of the higher number of molecules. When the concentration is equalised, the number of molecules moving in each direction is the same, resulting in no further net movement across the membrane. The lipid-soluble molecules dissolve into the phospholipid bi-layer and dissolve out into the intracellular fluid.

Facilitated diffusion

Large molecules that cannot pass through protein channels and are not lipid-soluble, particularly large sugars such as glucose, are picked up by a carrier. The combined glucose-carrier has a different chemical make-up, becomes lipid soluble and is therefore able to be dissolved through the phospholipid bilayer.

Active processes

Channels

Certain solutes are believed to activate a receptor in the integral protein channels. The channels take in the solute and expel it on the other side of the membrane in two stages. In the first stage the channel changes shape to open to receive the molecule. The second stage involves the outer end of the channel closing and the inner end opening, freeing the molecule into the cell. This process occurs in both directions. (See also the sodium - potassium pump under nervous tissue) The pump process can be used to transport substances against the concentration gradient.

Endocytosis & phagocytosis

The cell membrane first actively encloses the substance to be ingested, then the enclosure is taken into the cell as an envelope and opened. This process is used to take large items, such as bacteria and very large proteins either way across the cell membrane.

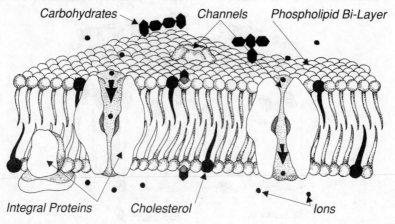

Figure   1-2 The Cell Membrane

Tissues

Simple epithelium

Squamous or pavement epithelium

This tissue comprises a single layer of flattened cells. It provides a smooth, thin, inactive lining to organs, including the heart, blood vessels, alveoli and lymphatic vessels.

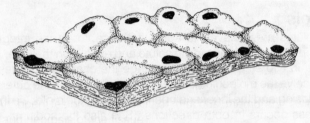

Figure   1-3

Ciliated epithelium

Cylindrical cells with minute hair-like processes, called cilia, on their free edge. The function of the cilia is to perform a sweeping movement, in one direction only, to waft mucus, dust and other small particles towards the pharynx. Forms the lining of the nose, larynx, trachea, bronchi. It is also found in the uterine tubes, where it assists in propelling the ovum towards the uterus.

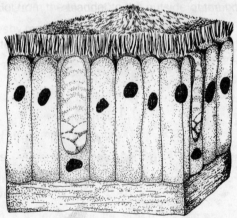

Figure   1-4

Compound Epithelium

Stratified epithelium

The deepest cells of this tissue are columnar, with superficial cells flattened. The tissue is found where there is a great deal of friction, such as the conjunctiva of the eye, the epidermis of the skin, the lining of the mouth, the lining of the pharynx, and the lining of the oesophagus. As the superficial cells are worn away, the lower cells migrate to the surface, flattening as they move upwards.

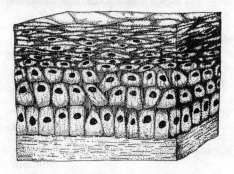

Figure   1-5

Transitional epithelium

Consisting of several layers of pear-shaped cells, the superficial layer of which may be flattened. Found in the pelvis of the kidney, the lining of the ureters and the lining of the urinary bladder.

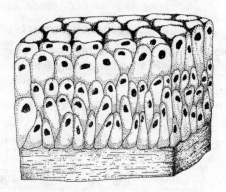

Figure   1-6

Connective tissues

Connective tissue is supportive tissue connecting more active tissue into functional units. The matrix may be semi-solid, jelly-like, or dense and rigid, depending on the position and function of the tissue.

Areolar tissue

Areolar tissue is an elastic tissue that connects and supports organs e.g.:- Under the skin for pliability, between muscles, supporting blood vessels and nerves. It is found in the submucous coat in the digestive tract and also in the interior of organs, binding together their main structure.

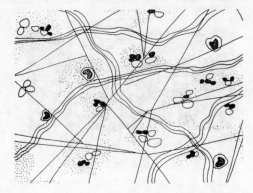

Figure   1-7

Adipose tissue

Fat cells supporting organs such as kidneys & eyes. It is also found between bundles of muscle fibres under the skin, which gives the body its smooth contours.

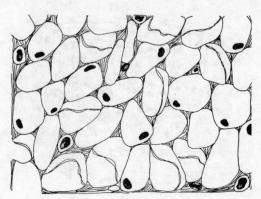

Figure   1-8

White fibrous tissue

Forms the ligaments binding bones. Protective covering of bone (periosteum). Protective outer covering of some organs e.g. kidneys, lymphatic glands, blood vessels and brain. Forming sheaths of muscles (muscle fascia).

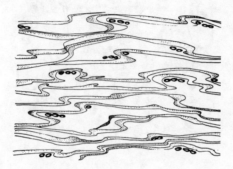

Figure   1-9

Yellow Elastic Tissue

Yellow elastic tissue is capable of considerable extension and recoil. It is found where a rapid change of shape is required e.g. the arteries, trachea, bronchi and lungs.

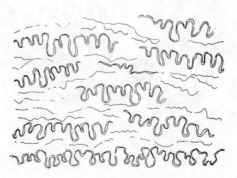

Figure   1-10

Lymphoid tissue

Lymphoid tissue is not a continuous tissue, but rather a collection of specialised cells known as lymphocytes. They are found in lymph, the fluid that circulates in the lymphatic system of nodes, spleen, tonsils, adenoids and appendix.

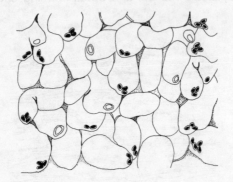

Figure   1-11

Blood

Blood is classed as a tissue as it is a collection of cells, specialised to perform a task or tasks. It comprises plasma (the liquid part) and formed elements (erythrocytes, leucocytes etc)

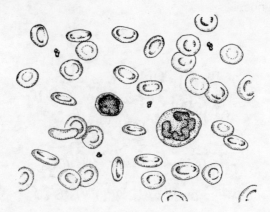

Figure   1-12

Skeletal muscle tissue

Skeletal muscle is voluntary muscle and is under the control of the somatic nervous system.

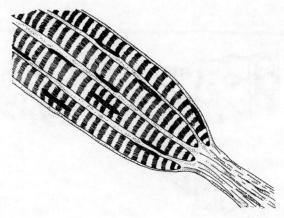

Figure   1-13

Cardiac Muscle

Although broadly similar to skeletal muscle, cardiac muscle is found only in the heart. It is capable of self-excitation and automaticity, but is heavily influenced by the autonomic nervous system, which alters the rate and power of the contractions.

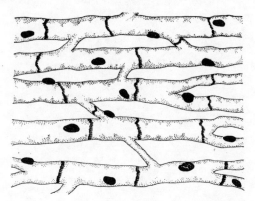

Figure   1-14

Smooth muscle

Smooth muscles are entirely under the control of the autonomic nervous system and are found in areas such as around arterioles and bronchioles, controlling diameter etc.

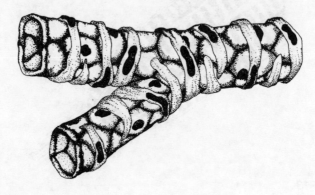

Figure   1-15

Organisation

Cavities of the body

The body can be divided into cavities which contain major organs. These are:
1. The cranial cavity 2. The thoracic cavity 3. The abdomino-pelvic cavity

The cranial cavity is bounded by the bones of the cranium and contains the brain and it's associated nerves and blood vessels. The vertebral canal is considered to be part of the cranial cavity and contains the spinal cord.

The thoracic cavity, or chest, is bounded by the rib cage and the diaphragm and contains the lungs and the mediastinum. The mediastinum is a large mass of tissues in the chest that contains the heart, the trachea, the left and right main bronchi, the oesophagus, the thymus gland, large blood vessels such as the aorta and vena cava and large lymphatic vessels.

The abdomino-pelvic cavity is bounded by the diaphragm and the pelvis. There is no clear boundary between the two parts. The upper part, the abdominal cavity, contains the stomach, the liver, the gall bladder, the spleen, the pancreas, the small intestine and most of the large intestine. The lower part, the pelvic cavity, contains the organs of reproduction, the remainder of the large intestine and the bladder and ureters.

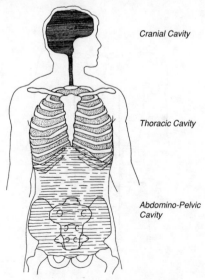

Cranial Cavity

Thoracic Cavity

Abdomino-Pelvic
Cavity

Figure   1-16

Abdominal regions

The abdominal cavity can be divided into nine regions, which can be used to locate the organs, although many of the organs overlap different regions. The horizontal demarcation lines between the regions are just below the ribcage and at the top of the pelvis. The vertical demarcation lines are in line with the midpoints of the clavicles.

The regions are named and located as follows:

Right Hypochondriac	Epigastric	Left Hypochondriac
Right Lumbar	Umbilical	Left Lumbar
Right Iliac	Hypogastric	Left Iliac

It is sometimes more convenient to divide the abdomino-pelvic cavity into quadrants, centred on the umbilicus, called the right and left upper and right and left lower quadrants, but this is much less precise.

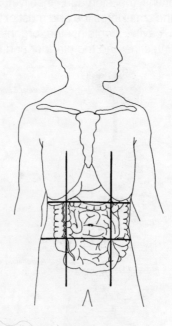

Figure   1-17

Biochemistry

Atomic structure & Electrolytes

Gas management & pH balance

Fluid management

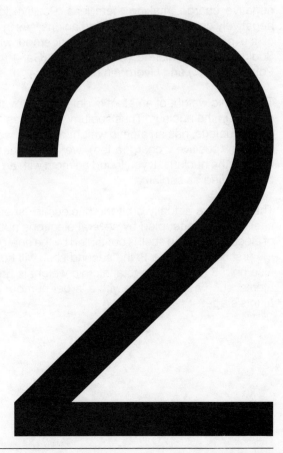

Atomic Structure

Atoms are made up of a nucleus and electrons which orbit the nucleus. These electrons are held in orbit by energy inherent in the atom. The nucleus is made up of protons, which have a positive (+) charge and neutrons, which have no charge. The electrons are negatively (-) charged.

An atom that has the same number of electrons as protons is electrically neutral, because the charges balance out. When an atom has an unequal number of protons and electrons, the atom has an overall positive or negative charge and is called an ion. Ionising radiation is so-called because it consists of high energy and highly active particles radiated from a substance (a radioactive isotope) that knock electrons out of orbit or knock protons out of the nucleus They can leave normally uncharged particles with a positive or negative charge, making them ions. Positive ions are called cations and negatively charged ions are called anions. (As in cathode and anode). Some of the principal ions that we are concerned with in body chemistry are:- Sodium (Na^+), Chloride (Cl^-), Calcium (Ca^{2-}) (has an extra 2 $^-$ charges), Potassium (K^+) and Hydrogen (H^+).

The atomic weight of an atom is determined by the number of neutrons and protons in the nucleus. Thus sodium, which has 11 neutrons and 12 protons in the nucleus, has an atomic weight of 23. As we know that sodium (Na^+) is a cation (positively charged ion), we know that there must be 13 electrons orbiting the nucleus. If you found an atom with an atomic weight of 23 it could be identified as sodium.

The electrons actually orbit the nucleus in "shells" or energy levels. These shells can be occupied by several electrons at the same time. The number of electrons in each shell is controlled by the energy level of the shell. Normally the first shell will hold 2, the second shell will hold 8, and the third shell will also hold 8 (or 18 if the total atomic weight is greater than 20). The heavier atoms, such as Plutonium, with a larger number of shells do not concern us at this stage.

Chemical reactions

Atoms possess kinetic energy, which holds the electrons in orbit around the nucleus and makes them vibrate, known as Brownian motion. (Some atoms vibrate at a frequency in the order of 30,000 Hz, or cycles per second). As the atoms vibrate, they are constantly colliding with other atoms. This is the means by which chemical reactions take place and also diffusion and osmosis take place (more later in fluid management). The rate of vibration increases with higher temperature, as heat is energy and energy is required to make the atoms vibrate. Chemical reactions therefore take place at a higher rate when the substances are heated.

Atoms that have a deficiency of two or three electron are liable, on colliding with another atom, to take an electron from an atom which has a surplus. The more electrons that are deficient, the more force is available in the shell to take and hold an electron from another atom. At the same time, the less electrons that are surplus, the more easily the atom will give it up to another atom, as it takes less energy to move one electron than move seven electrons. The deficiency or surplus determines the reactivity of the element. If there are no electrons surplus or deficient, the atom is inert, as it is difficult for it to form bonds or to lose or gain an electron.

Atoms can also share electrons, with the electron effectively orbiting both atoms at the same time. When this happens, the atoms are bonded, and they form a molecule, as in oxygen, which is normally found as a molecule of two atoms of oxygen bonded together, hence the chemical symbol O_2. When oxygen combines with hydrogen to form water, (H_2O) the oxygen atom shares an electron with the two hydrogen atoms. Atoms can also bond with atoms of a different element, so forming compounds, such as Sodium Chloride (NaCl) As sodium is positively charged and chloride is negatively charged, when they combine as sodium chloride the two charges balance out and the molecule is electrically neutral. Remember that an atom that loses or gains an electron during a chemical reaction can become charged, either negatively when gaining an electron or positively when losing an electron, but only if this results in an imbalance of charges.

The ability to combine chemically with other atoms is equal to the number of deficient or surplus electrons. What happens is that if an atom that is deficient in electrons comes close to an atom that has a surplus of electrons, the surplus electron jumps to the other atom or the two atoms combine and share an electron thereby making a molecule. Which of these happens depends on the individual characteristics of each atom. Note that the atom would only change into a different atom if the number of protons or neutrons changes. This only happens with nuclear fusion or fission which we will not attempt in the classroom.

Chemical reactions occur if there is a making or breaking of bonds between atoms. The release of energy causes the release of heat. (Hence the ability of the body to make heat by chemical reactions involving the breaking down of food in the cells). Conversely, the building up of molecules by the body requires energy, which is obtained when food is broken down. During a chemical reaction the number of atoms remains the same but the molecules are rearranged in bonding. These molecules have different properties due to the atoms having changed electron shells and therefore the ability to combine with different atoms.

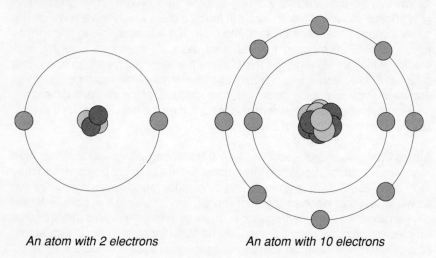

An atom with 2 electrons   *An atom with 10 electrons*

Figure 2-18

Chemicals referred to in this chapter are as follows:

Potassium **K** Carbon Dioxide **CO$_2$**
Water **H$_2$O** Bicarbonate **HCO$_3$**
Chloride **Cl** Iron **Fe** Calcium **Ca**
Sodium Bicarbonate **NaHCO$_3$**
Oxygen **O$_2$** Hydrogen **H**

Acids and pH

Acids have hydrogen in their make-up. The acidity of a fluid is determined by the proportion of free hydrogen ions (H^+) in the fluid. The alkalinity of a fluid is determined by the concentration of hydroxl ions (OH^-) in the fluid. The pH number is a fraction representing the proportion of H^+ ions in the solution It is derived from the scientific notation of the fraction. That is, if there is one hydrogen ion in 10,000 other atoms or 1×10^{-4} (this is 1×10 to the power of -4). The pH is then said to be 4. If there were one in 1,000,000 (1×10^{-6}) this would be equivalent to pH 6. A solution that has a pH greater than 7 is alkaline, a solution of pH less than 7 is acidic. A solution of pH 7 is neutral.

As 1 in 10,000 ($1 : 10^{-4}$) is a stronger concentration than 1 in 1,000,000 ($1 : 10^{-6}$) the pH of 4 is more acidic than pH of 6. A change in the pH of a whole number therefore signifies a change in concentration of ten fold over the previous number. The pH scale runs from 0 to 14, with 7 being neutral in chemistry terms. In bodily terms, however, the normal pH is about 7.35, with any change from this figure deemed to be acidosis or alkalosis.

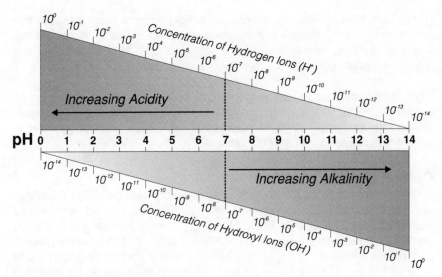

Figure 2-19 The pH Scale

Gas Management

Oxygen transport

100ml of blood holds a total of 20ml of oxygen (O_2). Of this total, only 3% is dissolved in the plasma, (as oxygen does not easily dissolve into water), and 97% is held on the hæmoglobin of the erythrocytes as oxyhæmoglobin. Hæmoglobin (Hb) is made up of a protein called globin and a pigment called heme. Heme is four combined atoms of iron (Fe), each of which is capable of holding one molecule of oxygen. The higher the partial pressure of oxygen in the blood, (PO_2) the more the hæmoglobin will hold, until it is fully saturated with one oxygen molecule to each heme molecule. Hæmoglobin picks up nearly a full load of oxygen even when the PO_2 is as low as 60 mmHg. (the normal partial pressure is 105mm Hg in oxygenated blood).There are several methods whereby an additional oxygen requirement is met more easily because of the physical conditions that the requirement causes.

When deoxygenated blood reaches the alveolar capillaries, PO_2 rises due to the oxygen being diffused down the concentration gradient from the atmosphere and hæmoglobin picks up a full load of oxygen. However, in the tissue capillaries, PO_2 in the intercellular fluid is low, causing the oxygen to disassociate in order to diffuse down the concentration gradient.

High acidity (low pH) causes the oxygen to split off more easily because the presence of free H^+ cations attracts the oxygen molecules. In this way, if the blood is acidotic, which arises from asphyxia among other causes, the oxygen splits off more easily and is available for use.

High temperature splits off oxygen more easily due to the presence of available energy, so that where the active cells, which require more oxygen, are warmer, the oxygen splits off more easily. Also DPG is given off by working cells which causes O_2 to split off more easily.

Carbon Dioxide transport

100ml of deoxygenated blood carries 4ml of carbon dioxide (CO_2). 7% of this is directly dissolved in the plasma as CO_2, 23% is carried attached to hæmoglobin as carbaminohæmoglobin (CO_2 is carried on the globin and O_2 on the heme part of the hæmoglobin). 70% is carried dissolved in the plasma as the bicarbonate anion ($HCO3^-$). When disposal of carbon dioxide (a waste product of cell metabolism) is required, a reaction takes place, the direction of which depends on the conditions present. Carbon dioxide leaves the cell and reacts with extracellular water to form carbonic acid.

The carbonic acid either dissociates into carbon dioxide and water (CO_2 and H_2O) or into hydrogen ions and bicarbonate (H^+ and $HCO3^-$)

$$CO_2 + H_2O <\ > H_2CO_3 <\ > H^+ + HCO_3^-$$

As CO_2 enters the plasma, Chloride (Cl^-) anions go from the plasma into the red cells in a process called the chloride shift. This maintains the ionic balance and is caused by electrolysis. Cl^- moving into the red cells combines with K^+ to form KCl (Potassium chloride). HCO_3 moving into the plasma combines with Na^+ cations to form $NaHCO_3$ (Sodium bicarbonate).

As will be seen, although O_2 can reach a saturation level, CO_2 does not, so acidosis can become worse and worse unless something is done about it. Chemical receptors in the body constantly monitor the pH of the body fluids. When they detect even a small change from the normal pH value of 7.35 they bring into effect systems to re-establish the balance. The fastest system is the buffer system. Chemicals that neutralise acids are secreted into the blood to quickly adjust the pH. This happens within seconds.

If this is insufficient a second system comes into play, the respiratory system. The respiratory system takes two to three minutes to have an appreciable effect on the blood pH. Raised rates of lung ventilation remove large amounts of CO_2 and water vapour (H_2O) from the blood by diffusion to the lower concentrations found in the atmosphere. This CO_2 is produced by breaking down H_2CO_3 (carbonic acid) into H_2O and CO_2. This raises the pH and thereby reduces the acidosis. If the rate of breathing is lowered the CO_2 is not released from the H_2CO_3 and therefore as the body is producing CO_2 from the metabolism, the CO_2 level and therefore the carbonic acid level builds up causing a lowering of the pH and therefore acidosis.

If this is still insufficient, a third system starts to work, the urinary system. The kidneys can excrete H^+ cations through the urine to reduce the concentration of free hydrogen ions in the blood. This process however takes several hours to days to make adjustments and is therefore the final backup system. Under normal circumstances, the three systems work together to maintain the pH balance.

Fluid management

The velocity of blood flow is slowest in the capillary network. This allows the exchange of gases, water, nutrients and wastes between the capillary blood and the interstitial fluid to take place. The exchanges take place down pressure gradients, and down concentration gradients due to osmosis (the net movement of water across any semi-permeable membrane) and diffusion (the net movement of solutes across a semi-permeable membrane).

The arterial blood has a hydrostatic pressure push (BHP) of about 30mm Hg and an osmotic pressure pull (BOP) of about 28mm Hg. The interstitial fluid has a hydrostatic pressure (IFHP) of about 0mm Hg and an osmotic pressure (pull) (IFOP) of about 6mm Hg. This results in a net outflow of fluid from the capillaries to the tissues, taking dissolved nutrients and gases with it.

At the venous end of the capillary bed, the blood hydrostatic pressure (BHP) is about 15mm Hg and the blood osmotic pressure (BOP) is about 28mm Hg. The interstitial fluid has a hydrostatic pressure (IFHP) of 0mm Hg and an osmotic pressure (pull) (IFOP) of about 6mm Hg. This results in a net outflow of fluid from the tissues to the capillaries, taking dissolved wastes and gases with it.

The lymph capillaries have a hydrostatic pressure of -1mm Hg whilst the interstitial fluid has a hydrostatic pressure of 0mm Hg, ensuring the drainage of the interstitial space.

There is a net pressure gradient of 8mm Hg from the arterial capillary blood to the interstitial fluid and 7mmHg pressure gradient from the interstitial fluid to the venous blood capillary. These pressures are the net result of several opposing forces due to the blood and interstitial fluid physical pressure (hydrostatic pressure) and the osmotic pull of the proteins and ions in the blood and interstitial fluid (osmotic pressure). All these pressures result in a flow of water and solutes from the arterial capillaries across the cells and into the venous capillaries. Should the balance of salts or proteins be altered, this may result in oedema of the tissues due to water retention or dehydration due to excessive water loss.

The Endocrine System

General Arrangement & Functions

The Pancreas

The Adrenal Glands

The Thyroid Gland

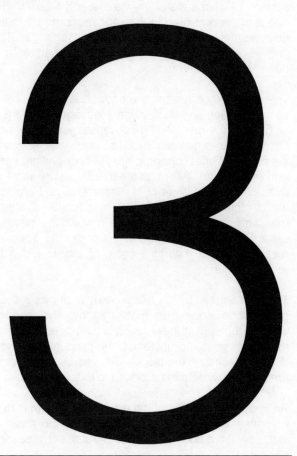

General arrangement

Function

The cells of the body operate in an internal environment which is closely controlled. If this environment were not controlled, the cells would not and could not carry out their functions. Each cell needs instructions to switch each of their many functions on and off at the correct time and in the correct sequence. For example, to move an arm, muscle cells need to be instructed to contract and at the same time, other cells need to be activated in the correct manner at the correct time in order to supply the muscle cell with its needs and to remove waste products.

The main task of co-ordination of the body is carried out by the nervous system, which measures the internal and external environment, assesses the needs of the body and then sends messages to individual cells or groups of cells via the nerves in order to carry out changes. These messages are sent in milliseconds, but they are limited to changes to specific cells supplied directly by the nerves.

There is another system, the endocrine system, (Gk Endo = within, Crine = secrete) which sends chemical messages to all the cells of the body at the same time, via the blood. These messages are hormones (Gk = start to work). Compared with nervous impulses, these messages take some time to reach the cells and effect change, but the changes are generally more long lasting and widespread. Although the messages are sent to all the cells at the same time, different cells react in different ways. Some cells do not react at all, whilst other cells perform different functions after receiving an identical message. This is due to the way in which the messages are received by the cells. Each cell has specific receptors for specific hormones and these receptors set in motion a chain of events within the cell to produce the required change.

These changes can be modified by changes in the internal environment in positive and negative feedback systems. The changes initiate other changes, which in turn, alter the secretion of hormones, either increasing or decreasing their production. For instance, the production of insulin is regulated by the level of glucose in the blood. The secretion of hormones is also affected by the nervous system in response to external stimuli.

An important function of the endocrine system is to initiate the fight-or-flight response to stressful events, such as personal danger or trauma. For instance, if the body is subject to trauma or blood loss, resulting in lowered

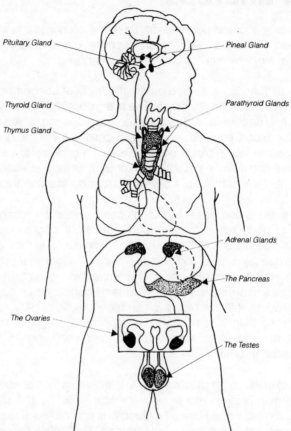

Figure 3-20   The Endocrine System

blood pressure, the adrenal glands secrete more adrenaline, which constricts blood vessels and makes the heart contract faster and harder to increase blood pressure. The results are measured by the nervous system and the adrenal glands are controlled to produce more or less adrenaline according to need.

The endocrine system is made up of several organs. The Pancreas, the Adrenal Glands, the Thyroid Gland, the Parathyroid Glands, The Pituitary Gland, The Ovaries and Testes, the Pineal Gland and the Thymus Gland. However, this chapter only covers the Pancreas, the Adrenal Glands and the Thyroid Gland.

The Pancreas

The pancreas is located posterior and slightly inferior to the stomach. The major portion of the pancreas is an exocrine gland concerned with the digestive system, which is not covered by this book.

The endocrine function is carried out by the Islets of Langerhans, which are clusters of cells within the pancreas. The Islets consist of three types of cells, alpha, beta and delta cells. Alpha cells secrete glucagon, which is a hormone used to raise blood glucose levels. Beta cells secrete insulin, which is a hormone used to lower blood glucose levels. Delta cells, secrete growth hormone inhibiting hormone, (GHIH), which inhibits the secretion of glucagon and insulin, thereby achieving a balance under normal conditions.

Glucagon acts to increase blood glucose levels by accelerating the conversion of glycogen in the liver into glucose. It also converts glycerol, amino acids and lactic acid into glucose. This glucose is then secreted into the blood to directly raise blood glucose levels. A negative feedback system controls the secretion of glucagon. The alpha cells detect the low level of blood glucose and are stimulated to secrete glucagon, which causes the liver to secrete glucose into the blood. When blood levels of glucose are raised, the cells are no longer stimulated and stop producing glucagon, thereby allowing blood levels of glucose to fall. Glucagon secretion is also inhibited by the secretion of GHIH.

Insulin acts to lower blood glucose levels. It facilitates the transport of glucose across cell membranes into skeletal muscle cells by the use of insulin receptors in the cell walls. Normally, glucose is not lipid-soluble and therefore is unable to pass through the cell membrane. The insulin receptors change the chemical make-up of the glucose, making it lipid-soluble. Insulin also accelerates the conversion of glucose into glycogen and its' subsequent deposition in the liver, it decreases the conversion of glycogen into glucose and decreases the conversion of glycerol, amino acids and lactic acid into glucose. Insulin secretion is also regulated by a negative feedback system, in which lowered blood glucose levels are detected by the beta cells and insulin production is decreased.

Insulin and glucagon therefore act in opposition to each other to maintain the normal blood levels of glucose, (3.5 - 5.7 mmol/l), whilst at the same time allowing for increases or decreases on demand for high energy requirements or digestion.

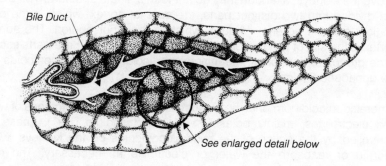

Bile Duct

See enlarged detail below

Figure 3-21 The Pancreas

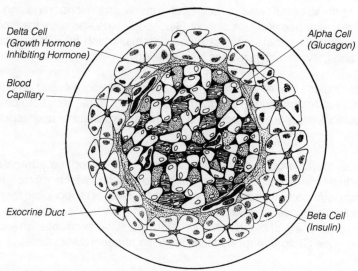

Delta Cell
(Growth Hormone
Inhibiting Hormone)

Blood
Capillary

Exocrine Duct

Alpha Cell
(Glucagon)

Beta Cell
(Insulin)

Figure 3-22 The Islets of Langerhans

The Adrenal Glands

The adrenal glands are so named because they are situated immediately above the kidneys, although they do not form a single structure. The glands are divided into two distinct parts, the adrenal cortex, which is the outer portion, and the adrenal medulla, which is the inner portion. The adrenal cortex is the site of production of steroid hormones. The three parts secrete three groups of hormones, the mineralocorticoids, the glucocorticoids and the gonadocorticoids.

Mineralocorticoid hormones help control the cellular concentrations of water and electrolytes, mainly potassium (K^+) and sodium (Na^+). These are controlled by the action of the mineralocorticoids on the kidneys, which secrete or reabsorb the water or electrolyte as necessary. The main mineralocorticoid secreted by the adrenal cortex is aldosterone.

Glucocorticoids are concerned with the regulation of metabolic activity and available energy. Various methods are employed, usually in conjunction with other hormones. These include changing the rate of protein catabolisation, transportation of amino acids from cells to the liver and the conversion of amino acids into glucose, and conversion of fatty acids from adipose tissue, which releases the stored energy. The additional glucose can be used by the body to fight stressful events such as trauma, situations requiring a fight-or-flight response and lack of food. Glucocorticoids also raise the blood levels of substances that constrict blood vessels, which increases blood pressure and they also help reduce inflammation.

Gonadocorticoids are otherwise known as sex hormones and include œstrogen and testosterone, the main female and male sex hormones. Gonadocorticoids regulate activities such as ovulation and sperm production.

The adrenal medulla contains chromaffin cells, which produce adrenaline and noradrenaline. Adrenaline is a sympathomimetic, which mimics the effects of the sympathetic nervous system. This system is responsible for the fight-or-flight responses, such as increases in heart rate, increases in respiration and raising of blood pressure. Noradrenaline produces the same responses. (See Chapter 4 for details) (See also phaechromocytoma).

The Thyroid Gland

The thyroid gland is found immediately below the larynx, on either side of and anterior to the trachea. It secretes chemicals collectively known as the thyroid hormones. The hormones have three main functions, controlling the activity of the nervous system, regulating metabolism and energy levels, and regulating growth and development and .

The activity of the nervous system is controlled by changing the reactivity of neurons.

Regulation of metabolism is achieved by stimulating carbohydrate and lipid catabolism and increasing the rate of protein synthesis. This increase in catabolism has the net effect of increasing the overall metabolic rate.

Growth and development is particularly important in the early stages of life, when the thyroid hormones regulate the speed and areas of growth of tissues, particularly nervous tissue. Lack of thyroid hormones in fœtal life can lead to cretinism.

The Nervous System

Nerve Cells

Nerve Impulse Transmission

The Brain

The Spinal Cord

The Autonomic Nervous System

Reflex Actions

Cranial Nerves

General Arrangement

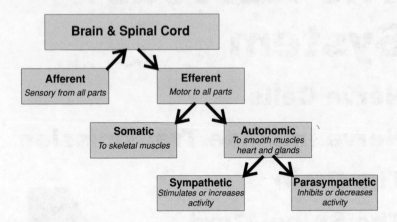

The nervous system can be divided into functional sections.

The Central Nervous System consists of the brain and spinal cord, which act as an integrative network, taking in information, processing it and giving out orders.

The Peripheral Nervous System consists of the Afferent and Efferent branches. The afferent transmits sensory information from all parts of the body to the brain. (It tells what is affecting the body). The efferent transmits motor commands to all parts of the body. (It has effects on the body).The efferent branch is divided into the Somatic and Autonomic systems.

The Somatic Nervous System is concerned with efferent transmissions to the skeletal muscles (under control of the will).

The Autonomic Nervous System is concerned with efferent transmissions to the smooth muscles, glands and the heart, which are not under control of the will.

The Autonomic system is divided into the Sympathetic and the Parasympathetic branches. The Sympathetic branch is concerned with efferent transmissions that (usually) stimulate or increase activity. The Parasympathetic branch is concerned with efferent transmissions that (usually) inhibit or decrease activity.

Nerve Cells

There are two main types of nerve cells, NEURONS and NEUROGLIA

Neurons

NEURONS are involved in the control and transmission of impulses. The different neurons may be classified by structure and function. The structural classification of neurons is based on the number of processes extending from the cell body.

MULTIPOLAR neurons have several dendrites and one axon. Most of the neurons in the brain and spinal cord are of this type.

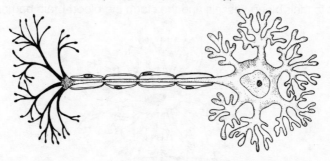

UNIPOLAR neurons have only one process extending from the cell body. This single process divides into a central branch, which functions as an axon and a peripheral branch, which functions as a dendrite They are found in the posterior root (sensory) ganglia of spinal nerves and the ganglia of cranial nerves that carry general somatic sensory impulses.

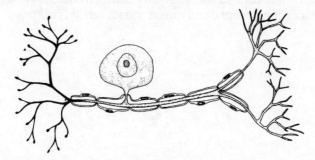

BIPOLAR neurons, which have one dendrite and one axon, are only found in the retina, inner ear and olfactory area and are not discussed here.

The functional classification of neurons is based on the direction that the nerve transmits the impulse.

SENSORY or AFFERENT neurons transmit from the nerve ending to the brain and from lower to higher centres in the central nervous system

Neuroglia

NEUROGLIA, or glial cells, (Greek Neuro = nerve, glia = glue) provide support, protection and nutrition to the whole system. They are subdivided into:

ASTROCYTES (Astro = star, cyte = cell) which are star shaped cells with numerous processes. They form a supporting network in the CNS, they attach neurons to their blood vessels and they form the blood-brain barrier.

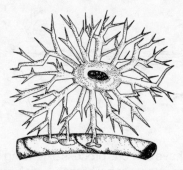

Figure 4-23 Astrocyte

OLIGODENDROCYTES (Greek oligo = few, dendro = tree) resemble astrocytes, but with fewer and shorter processes. They give support by forming semi-rigid connective tissue rows between neurons in the CNS. They also produces the phospholipid myelin sheath around neurons.

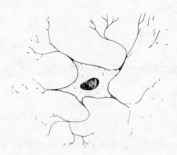

Figure 4-24 Oligodendrocyte

MICROGLIA (micro = small, glia = glue) They are small cells with few processes derived from monocytes, usually stationary, but can migrate to the site of injury. Also known as brain macrophages. (macro = large phage = eat)

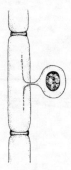

Figure 4-25 Microglia

EPENDYMA (Greek ependyma = upper garment) Epithelial cells arranged in a single layer and ranging in shape from squamous to columnar. Many are ciliated. They form an epithelial lining for the ventricles of the brain and the central canal of the spinal cord, assisting in the circulation of cerebro-spinal fluid.

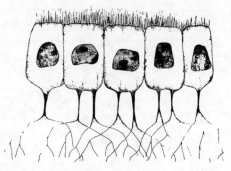

Figure 4-26 Ependyma

Neuron structure

All nerve cells have the same basic structure. Each is specialised in some way to perform specific functions, such as nerve cells in the eye and in the cerebrum.

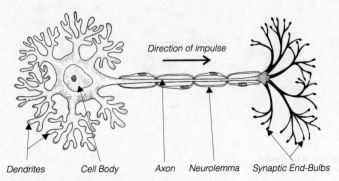

Figure 4-27 General Neuron Structure

The Cell body

The contents and structure of the cell body is much the same as other cells in the body, with various organelles performing their normal functions. A difference from other cells is that the neuron cell body puts out processes (the number of which depends on the type of neuron). These processes, formed from cytoplasmic proteins, form the axon and dendrites of the neuron.

Synaptic end-bulbs

The end of the neuron has synaptic end-bulbs, which contain the neurotransmitters which are released into the synaptic cleft (the small space between neurons and the effector organ or next neuron). The release is triggered by the change in the polarity of the axon at the end-bulb.

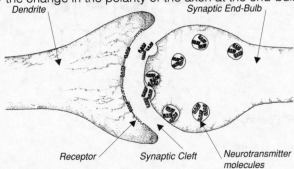

Figure 4-28 Synaptic End-Bulb

Dendrites

These are responsible for the collection of impulses from other neurons and from receptors in organs. They contain receptors which are sensitive to the neurotransmitters released from the synaptic end-bulbs of the preceding neuron.

The Axon

The axon is a multi-filament fibre, formed from cytoplasm, which transmits nerve impulses away from the cell body to another neuron or to a muscular or glandular receptor. The cytoplasm is surrounded by the axolemma, a plasma membrane. Nutrients to and waste products from the axon are transported to and from the cell body within the neurolemma and it also functions in the regeneration of damaged neurons (note that the neurolemma only occurs in neurons outside the central nervous system, which accounts for the fact that neurons within the central nervous system do not regenerate if damaged.

Most axons outside the central nervous system, and some within, are surrounded by a white phospholipid sheath known as the myelin sheath. The myelin sheath is formed from neurolemmocytes, glial cells which wrap themselves around the axon. It occurs as single cells, with a small gap, the Node of Ranvier between. The function of the myelin sheath is to increase the speed of nerve impulse conduction and to insulate and maintain the axon. The sheath insulates the outside of the axon from the electrical changes from adjacent parts of the same axon and allows the polarity change from one Node of Ranvier to affect the polarity of an adjacent Node of Ranvier, so that the impulse travels i□a series of rapid jumps, instead of a slow progression. The white matter of the spinal cord and brain is composed of myelinated neurons, whilst the grey matter is unmyelinated neurons. The myelin sheath is necessary in the peripheral nervous system due to the very long neurons, some of which reach one metre in length. If the neurons were unmyelinated, the impulses could take several seconds to reach their receptors.

Neurotransmitters

The main neurotransmitter in the central nervous system is acetylcholine (ACh). The effect of ACh is normally excitatory. The normal synaptic delay, caused by the time taken for the neurotransmitters to cross the synaptic cleft, is 1/500th of a second. ACh is inactivated by an enzyme called acetylcholinesterase and returned to the synaptic end-bulbs, ready for another nerve impulse. Noradrenaline is also a neurotransmitter, but is usually found in the autonomic nervous system

Nerve impulse transmission

Signals, or impulses, are transmitted along the neuron axons by the generation of an action potential, or wave of electrical negativity, which runs along the membrane of the nerve cell axon. This wave is propagated by the movement of sodium and potassium ions (Na^+ and K^+) in and out of the cell.

At rest, the neuron has 30 times more potassium (K^+) inside than outside and 14 times as much sodium (Na^+) outside than inside. It also has a large number of negatively charged protein molecules inside the cell, which are too large to be diffused through the cell membrane. K^+ and Na^+ are constantly being pumped into and out of the cell by the actions of diffusion and active transport channels. (See cells and tissues). The cell membrane is 100 times more permeable to the outflow of K^+ than Na^+ and the channels pump 3 times as much Na^+ out than K^+ in. The Na^+ is entering the cell by diffusion, but is then pumped out at three times the rate. The K^+ is being pumped in, but is diffusing out at 100 times the rate. This results in the cell membrane having a difference of charge (electrical potential) between the inside and outside, with the outside being predominantly positive and the inside being predominantly negative. The cell is said to be polarised.

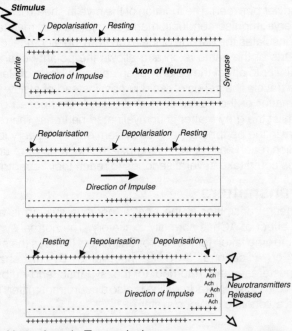

Figure 4-29 Nerve Impulse Transmission

The purpose of the sodium-potassium (Na^+ / K^+) pump is to maintain that imbalance of electrical charges. This allows a threshold stimulus, (one that is strong enough to be over the threshold that will depolarise the cell), to change the electrical potential of the cell membrane, in a wave of negativity, which can be propagated down the axon and effect a change at the synaptic end-bulb and therefore activate the muscle or cells at the end.

A threshold stimulus (electrical, chemical or mechanical) changes the cell membranes permeability to Na^+ by opening additional, voltage sensitive Na^+ channels. As the Na^+ floods into the cell, due to the increased permeability of the cell membrane, the internal charge changes to more positive and the external charge changes to more negative (in relation to one another). This is depolarisation and is achieved within 1/10,000th of a second.

The wave of change in polarity of the cell spreads along the length of the cell because the change instigates the opening of the voltage sensitive channels in adjoining areas of the cell membrane. This instigates an action potential. The K^+ then begins to flow out through the normal diffusion process and also through K^+ channels that are activated by the action potential, and the electrical potential begins to change back. This is "repolarisation". Until the cell is repolarised, the generation of a fresh action potential is impossible.

As the K^+ ions flow back out, the cell becomes hyperpolarised for a time, until the sodium-potassium pump has operated sufficiently to convert the membrane electrical potential back to its normal resting state.

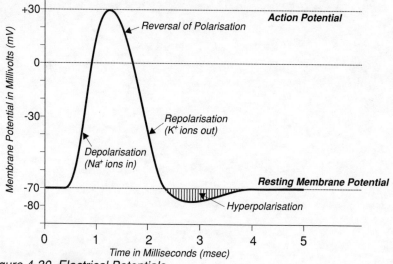

Figure 4-30 Electrical Potentials

During this hyperpolarisation, the cell is in the relative refractory period, when a very strong stimulus will generate an action potential. All this happens in a very short space of time. Large nerve fibres can conduct up to 2,500 impulses (stimuli) per second (1 every 0.4 msec), due to their large surface area and the large capacity of ions. Small fibres can only conduct 250 per second (1 every 4.0 msec).

An excessive number of stimuli in a very short time will result in no action potential being generated because of the massive ionic shift taking place. The cell simply runs out of ions to shift in order to achieve depolarisation.

When the impulse reaches the synapse, (the join between nerve cells that allows transmission), neurotransmitters are released from the presynaptic end-bulb of one nerve cell and released into the synaptic cleft (the space between the neurons). The neurotransmitters link into specific receptors in the dendrite of the postsynaptic neuron which then continue the transmission of the impulse to the nerve ending.

THE BRAIN

The brain in an average adult is made up of about 1,000 billion neurons and is one of the largest organs of the body, weighing about 1300 grams (3lbs). The brain consists of grey matter and white matter. In simple terms, the grey matter is unmyelinated neurons and the white matter is myelinated neurons.

The principal parts of the brain are the cerebrum, the cerebellum, the mid-brain, the pons and the medulla oblongata.

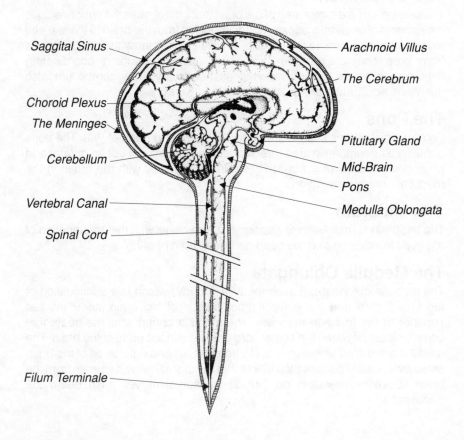

Figure 4-31 The Brain and Spinal Cord

The Cerebrum

The cerebrum is where the coordination of all conscious thought takes place, the seat of the intellect.

The Brain Stem

The Brain Stem consists of three parts:The pons (bridge) lies directly above the medulla and anterior to the cerebellum. It is mainly a connection between the various parts of the brain, with transverse fibres from the cerebellum and longitudinal fibres which connect the spinal cord or medulla with the upper parts of the brain stem.

The Cerebellum

The cerebellum is a motor area of the brain that coordinates the subconscious movements of skeletal muscles. Motor impulses from the brain to the skeletal muscles are also sent to the cerebellum, which compares them with results from proprioceptors on the joints and muscles, sending coordinating impulses to adjust the movements as necessary. The cerebellum also maintains equilibrium and posture in the same way.

The Pons

Some cranial nerves arise in the pons; (V, VI, VII and parts of VIII). The pons contains a pneumotaxic area (greek pneumo = air, taxic = speed or rate) and an apneuistic area (a = none) These areas, together with the areas in the medulla, control respiration.

The Midbrain

The midbrain is mainly a relay station but also deals with the coordination of the eyes from vision and the head and trunk from hearing.

The Medulla Oblongata

The medulla oblongata, (Greek medulla = body) which is a continuation of the spinal cord and forms the inferior portion of the brain stem, lies just superior to the foramen magnum. The medulla contains all the tracts that communicate between the spinal cord and the various parts of the brain. The medulla is the area where the nerves from the left and right sides of the brain cross over, called decussation. (Note that the cranial nerves all arise from the brain above the decussation, but all the spinal nerves arise below the decussation.)

Vital Centres

Within the medulla are three vital centres. The cardiac centre regulates the rate of the heart and the force of contraction, the medullary rhythmicity centre adjusts the basic rhythm of breathing and the vasomotor centre regulates the diameter of blood vessels. These centres will be discussed within their relevant system chapters.

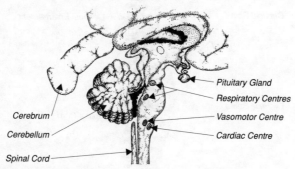

Cerebrum
Cerebellum
Spinal Cord

Pituitary Gland
Respiratory Centres
Vasomotor Centre
Cardiac Centre

Figure 4-32 The Vital Centres

The medulla also contains the origins of several pairs of cranial nerves (parts of VIII, all of IX, X, XI and XII). There are connections to the cerebellum which ensure the efficiency of voluntary movements, especially precision movements.

The Diaencephalon

The Diencephalon consists of two main parts,

The Thalamus

The Thalamus (gk thalamos = inner chamber) is 80% of the diencephalon and it interprets pain, temperature, touch, light and pressure and relays information between all parts of the brain and the spinal cord.

The Hypothalamus

The Hypothalamus is a small part of the diencephalon but it controls, coordinates and integrates the autonomic nervous system,receives and integrates sensory impulses from the viscera. It is the principal intermediary between the nervous system and the endocrine system. It is the centre for psychosomatic impulses It controls normal body temperature. It is responsible for the sensation of hunger and thirst and also fullness. It maintains the waking state and sleep patterns and is believed to be the centre for the "body clock".

The Spinal Cord

The spinal cord is the nervous connection between the brain and the rest of the body. It also serves as the reflex centre by association neurons within the cord connecting sensory and motor nerves directly.

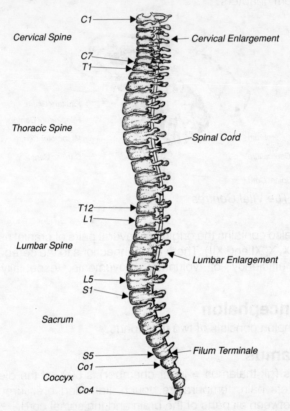

Figure 4-33 The Spinal Cord

The cord is divided into a series of 31segments, each giving rise to a pair of spinal nerves. Each individual spinal nerve consists of a sensory and a motor nerve. The pairs of nerves are named and numbered according to where they arise. There are 8 cervical, 12 thoracic, 5 lumbar, 5 sacral and 1 coccygeal. (The cranial nerves all arise in the cranium and do not form part of the spinal cord.) Some spinal nerves branch, rebranch and cross-connect to form a plexus. These are the cervical plexus (C1-C5), the brachial plexus (C5-T1), the lumbar plexus (L1-L4) and the sacral plexus (L4-S3). Spinal nerves T2-T12 are the intercostal (Thoracic) nerves.

The spinal cord is roughly cylindrical in shape, with a slight anterior to posterior flattening and it consists of both white matter and grey matter. The white matter is bundles of myelinated axons of motor and sensory neurons and forms the motor and sensory vertical tracts. The grey matter is primarily nerve cell bodies and the dendrites and unmyelinated axons of association and motor neurons.

The grey matter is formed into an H-shaped vertical column, which is divided functionally into regions called horns. There are the anterior, posterior and lateral grey horns. The lateral horns are present in the thoracic, upper lumbar and sacral segments of the cord. The spinal nerves arise from the posterior and anterior grey horns of the grey matter. The posterior root contains only sensory nerve fibres, the anterior root contains only motor fibres. The sensory and motor fibres leave the cord separately and join outside as one spinal nerve. The spinal nerves are therefore mixed nerves.

The cell bodies of the motor neurons are located in the grey matter of the spinal cord. If the motor neuron supplies a skeletal muscle, the cell bodies are located in the anterior grey horn. However, if the motor nerve supplies a smooth muscle, cardiac muscle or gland within the autonomic nervous system, the cell bodies are located in the lateral grey horn. The cell bodies of sensory neurons are located outside the cord in the posterior root ganglion. The association neurons are situated in the lateral grey horns and serve as connections between the sensory and motor nerves in the reflex arc. (described later). In the centre of the grey matter is the central canal, which is a continuation of the subarachnoid space and contains cerebrospinal fluid. The central canal is lined with ciliated ependyma.

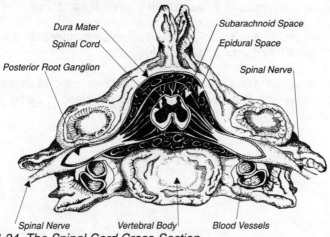

Figure 4-34 The Spinal Cord Cross-Section

The white matter is also divided into regions, called vertical columns, which consist of distinct bundles of myelinated fibres of sensory and motor nerves. The columns are further subdivided into tracts which are distinct bundles of axons. The ascending tracts are sensory and the descending tracts are motor.

The spinal cord begins as a continuation of the medulla oblongata and terminates about the level of the second lumbar vertebra. At this level it reduces to the conus medullaris (Gk= Cone shaped body). From the end of the conus a filament of pia mater called the filum terminale attaches to the coccyx. The cord is held in position laterally by other extensions of the pia mater, called denticulate ligaments, which extend outwards to attach to the dura mater.

The overall length of the cord is about 42-45 cm in adults and it has a diameter of approx 2.5 cm in the thoracic region. There are two thickenings of the cord, at the cervical region and the lumbar region, where the main nerves serving the upper and lower limbs enter and leave the cord. The cord is protected by the fact that it lies within the foramina of the vertebrae, which form a bony ring around the cord. It is also protected by the meninges, in the same way as the brain. The cord is also bathed in cerebrospinal fluid, which acts as a shock absorber and source of nutrition.

As the spinal cord is part of the central nervous system, the axons are not regenerated following damage. The spinal nerves, being part of the peripheral nervous system, do regenerate following damage.

For an axon to regenerate, it has to satisfy several conditions:
1. The cell body must be intact.
2. The fibres must be in association with neurolemmocytes (Schwann cells)
3. Scar tissue formation should not be too rapid.

However, research is under way into the actual process of axon regeneration (using goldfish and frog optic nerves), and progress is being made into persuading CNS axons to regenerate.

The Meninges

The meninges (singular: meninx) are the three coverings that surround the brain and spinal cord.

The outer meninx is the Dura Mater, which, in the brain, is a thick, dense, inelastic fibrous membrane composed of two parts. The outer layer, which forms the periosteum of the interior of the skull, is tough, rough textured and fibrous and follows the shape of the skull exactly.

The inner layer is a smooth membrane primarily made up of epithelium and is generally closely allied to the outer layer. However, the two layers separate to form the cerbral sinuses, which provide drainage for the cerebrospinal fluid to be returned to the cardiovascular system. (More on that later.) The spinal cord dura mater consists only of the inner smooth layer. The inner surface of the vertebral column is lined with a layer of fat and connective tissue, interspersed with blood vessels. This provides rather more protection for the spinal cord than the meninges alone.

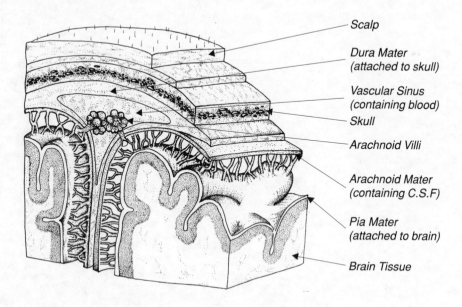

Scalp

Dura Mater
(attached to skull)

Vascular Sinus
(containing blood)

Skull

Arachnoid Villi

Arachnoid Mater
(containing C.S.F)

Pia Mater
(attached to brain)

Brain Tissue

Figure 4-35 The Meninges

The middle meninx is the Arachnoid Mater (Greek Arachne = spiders web), so called because the sub-arachnoid space is filled with a dense web of fibres, which separate it from the Pia Mater.

Between the dura mater and the arachnoid mater is a potential space, filled with serous fluid. The arachnoid mater is a delicate membrane that surrounds the brain and spinal cord, but is separated from it by the sub-arachnoid space and the pia mater. The sub-arachnoid space is filled with cerebrospinal fluid, which is described later.

The inner meninx, which is directly attached to the surface of the brain, is the Pia Mater (Greek = delicate mother). The pia mater forms the outer surface of the brain, consisting of a very fine plexus of blood vessels held together by an extremely fine areolar tissue.

Cerebro-Spinal Fluid

The brain and spinal cord are surrounded by cerebro-spinal fluid (CSF). The functions of this clear, colourless fluid are to provide nourishment, waste disposal, support and cushioning.

CSF is a clear, colourless fluid, which contains glucose, proteins, urea, salts and lymphocytes. Glucose is the main nutrient for the brain and spinal cord, as most other substances are trapped by the blood-brain barrier, whilst proteins, urea, and salts are necessary for cell growth and repair. The lymphocytes perform their normal role of infection control. The subarachnoid space contains between approximately 80 and 150ml of CSF

CSF is formed by filtration from the blood and secretion by the ependymal cells of the necessary components in the choroid plexuses in the ventricles of the brain. The majority is made in the lateral ventricles, from where it passes to the third ventricle, where more is added. It then passes into the fourth ventricle and thence into the subarachnoid space at the rear of the brain and spinal cord. It circulates down the posterior subarachnoid space of the spinal cord and back up the anterior space around the spinal cord and brain.

Used CSF is then reabsorbed into the venous system in the superior saggital sinus, through the arachnoid villi, which line the sinus. Arachnoid villi are projections of the arachnoid mater, which filter the CSF.

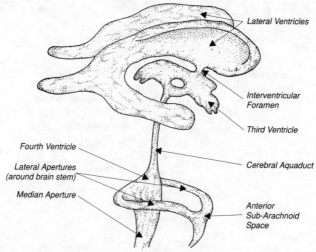

Figure 4-36 The Ventricles of the Brain

The Autonomic Nervous System

The Autonomic Nervous System is also known as the visceral efferent nervous system, as its function is generally entirely efferent (motor) and its effects are only on the viscera, (such as the heart, lungs and digestive system etc), not the skeletal muscles.

The system has two effects, excitatory and inhibitory. The excitatory part is the sympathetic branch and the inhibitory part is the parasympathetic branch. This applies in general terms, not absolute terms, as some effects are excitatory, depending on the organ, such as the wall of the urinary bladder. The main effects of the two branches are characterised by the sympathetic system being the fight and flight system and the parasympathetic being the rest and repose system.

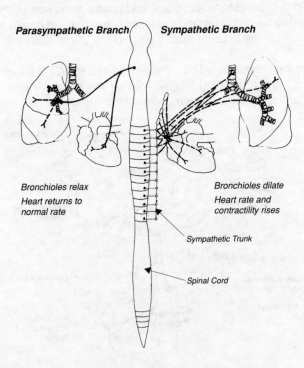

Parasympathetic Branch **Sympathetic Branch**

Bronchioles relax
Heart returns to
normal rate

Bronchioles dilate
Heart rate and
contractility rises

Sympathetic Trunk

Spinal Cord

Figure 4-37 The Autonomic Nervous System

The effects of the system on various organs are too numerous and diverse to list here fully. In general, they are that the sympathetic system prepares the body for action, by such effects as dilating the lungs to gain more oxygen, raising the pulse rate to achieve more circulation of that oxygen and peripheral vasoconstriction to divert that increased blood flow to the skeletal muscles and vital organs such as the brain. It also has less obvious effects, such as mobilising more glucose from the liver and conversion of fats to glycogen. The parasympathetic branch, which usually dominates unless the body or emotions are under stress, has the effects that are required for repair and recharging the body. The blood flow is changed back to normal, (there is no vasodilation caused by the parasympathetic branch). The digestive system starts to work, to convert food into proteins and fat stores, the bladder is more easily emptied and the sex organs are able to be utilised.

The parasympathetic branch arises in the mid-brain, pons and medulla (the brain stem) and the 2nd to 4th sacral vertebrae. The brain stem part innervates the pupils, the nose and tear glands, the heart, lungs, the liver, the G.I. tract and the kidneys. The sacral part innervates the ureters, the urinary bladder, the rectum and the sex organs. The sympathetic branch innervates all the same organs, but arises from the thoracic vertebrae and the 1st and 2nd lumbar vertebrae. The nerves all pass from the brain stem and spinal cord to ganglia, where they synapse with a second nerve to innervate the organs. (The somatic nervous system innervates the organs directly with one nerve.) The pre-ganglionic nerves are all myelinated and the post-ganglionic nerves are all non-myelinated. The ganglia for the parasympathetic branch are in or close to the effector organ, whilst the sympathetic branch ganglia are close to the spinal cord. This has the effect of making the myelinated (fast transmission) part of the nerves different lengths. This is thought to be because the sympathetic branch is assisted by adrenaline and therefore does not need myelination.

The neurotransmitter in the parasympathetic nervous system is Acetylcholine (ACh) and the main neurotransmitter in the sympathetic system is Noradrenaline (NE) (Some postganglionic sympathetic neurons use ACh where the effects are to be inhibitory, such as the GI tract). The sympathetic neurotransmitter (NE) is also assisted by the production of adrenaline by the adrenal glands. This makes the effects of the sympathetic system more powerful and longer lasting. (Normally the parasympathetic branch dominates and a powerful effect is required to overcome it.) ACh is quickly destroyed, so the sympathetic system can quickly take over when necessary, whilst sympathetic stimulation takes a while to suppress due to the oceans of adrenaline floating about in the blood.

The general method of transmission and innervation is the same as for the somatic nervous system. The actual effect of the neurotransmitters is determined by the type of post-synaptic receptor with which it interacts. In the parasympathetic branch there are two types, muscarinic and nicotinic. The effects of the muscarinic receptors are inhibitory (muscarine is a poisonous mushroom which slows everything down) The nicotinic are excitatory (nicotine increases permeability of nerve cells and therefore speeds up nervous conduction and induces a state of nervous excitability). In the sympathetic branch there are also two types of receptor, alpha and beta (a and b) The effects of the alpha receptors is generally excitatory and the effects of beta receptors is generally inhibitory, (with some notable exceptions, such as the heart)

The effects on the various systems will be discussed within the different sections, as the operation of the respiratory and cardiovascular systems are controlled by the autonomic system. In general terms at rest the parasympathetic dominates, with input by the sympathetic to keep a balance and to provide enough energy to keep the body going. The main effects that we are concerned with are that under stress the sympathetic branch dilates the pupils; increases heart rate contraction and automaticity; constricts skin and visceral blood vessels; raises the respiratory rate; dilates the bronchioles; converts fat to glycogen and converts glycogen to glucose. The parasympathetic branch has the opposite effects. The effects of the system described are in general terms, the whole system is best studied with target organs in mind.

Reflex actions

Reflex actions are very rapid responses to certain stimuli in the external or internal environment that allow the body to maintain homeostasis and to protect itself.

Reflex actions are centred in the spinal cord. They require five parts to act.
1. A receptor to sense the change in environment.
2. A sensory neuron to transmit the information to the spinal cord.
3. A reflex centre to generate a motor impulse after receiving a sensory impulse. In the centre the impulse may be inhibited transmitted or rerouted.
4. A motor neuron to transmit the motor impulse to the target muscle gland or organ.
5. An effector which is the target organ muscle or gland which carries out the required response, such as muscle contraction or a decrease or increase in the secretion of a gland.

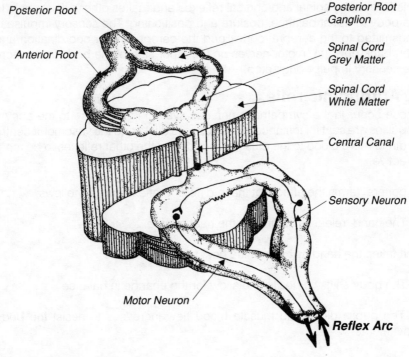

Figure 4-38 The Reflex Arc

There are four main types of reflex that concern the paramedic:

1. Spinal reflex

This action is the fastest and is composed of three parts. The sensory impulse is received from a sensory receptor. This is passed into the spinal cord and through an association neuron directly to a motor neuron where it passes to a motor effector. It is used where a protective action is immediately required, as when a hand is placed on a hot object.

2. Cortical reflex

This follows the spinal reflex and reinforces, modifies or inhibits it. The sensory impulse passes from the sensory nerve through the association neuron and is transmitted to the cerebral cortex for modification. It is then passed back down the cord to the appropriate motor neuron on the same side as the original sensory impulse.

3. Coordinating reflex

This follows the spinal and cortical reflexes and makes other adjustments to the body to assist balance, posture and positioning. The sensory impulse is transmitted to the cerebral cortex and the cerebellum for coordination and then back down to motor nerves on the other side of the body from where the sensory impulse originated.

4. Autonomic reflex

These occur in the sympathetic nervous system in response to the above. Impulses are sent for instance to the pupils to dilate and the vasomotor centre to direct more blood to the muscles in order for the other reflexes to be more effective.

In general terms the effects of these different reflexes are as follows:

1. The hand releases its grip on the heat source.

2. It takes the hand away from the heat source.

3. The body shifts its position to allow for the change in balance.

4. The pupils dilate and muscle blood flow increases to assist the body movements.

There are several other types of reflex, but these are are not discussed in full detail.

The stretch reflex (a monosynaptic reflex in which the sudden stretching of a muscle causes a contraction of that same muscle).

The tendon reflex (a polysynaptic reflex to protect the tendon against overstretching - related to the stretch reflex).

The flexor reflex (a protective reflex where flexor muscles are stimulated while extensor muscles are inhibited).

The crossed extensor reflex (where extension of the joints of one limb occurs in conjunction with contraction of the the flexor muscles of the opposite limb).

The Bainbridge reflex, (the increased heart rate following increased pressure in the right atrium).

The Babinski sign, (resulting from gentle stimulation of the outer margin of the sole of the foot. The great toe is extended (upwards), A positive Babinski sign after 18 months of age is considered abnormal and indicates a an interruption of the corticospinal tract, usually in the upper portion. The normal response after 18 months of age is the plantar reflex or negative Babinski sign, which is a curling under of all the toes, accompanied by a slight turning in and flexion of the anterior part of the foot.)

Cranial Nerves

There are 12 pairs of cranial nerves. 9 pairs originate in the brain stem, (The Olfactory, Optic and Auditory nerves arise in the olfactory area, the retina and the inner ear respectively) but all 12 pass through foramina in the cranium.

The cranial nerves are designated with Roman numerals as well as names. The Roman numerals indicate the order in which the nerves originate (from front to back) and the names indicate the distribution or function.

Some cranial nerves are sensory only, but the remainder are mixed motor and sensory. Although the mixed nerves contain both motor and sensory, they are primarily motor.

The cell bodies of sensory fibres lie outside the brain, but the cell bodies of motor fibres lie within nuclei in the brain. The cranial nerves are part of the somatic nervous system, but some of the nerve fibres belong to the autonomic nervous system. The reason they are described together is that some autonomic fibres are bundled together with somatic fibres as they leave the brain and spinal cord.

The Cranial Nerves

No	Name	Origin	Sensory Function	Motor Function
I	**Olfactory**	Nasal Mucosa	Smell	None
II	**Optic**	Retina	Vision	None
III	**Oculomotor**	Mid-brain	Proprioception of eye and eyelid	Movement of eye and eyelid. Accommodation of lens and constriction of pupil
IV	**Trochlear**	Mid-brain	Proprioception of eye	Movement of eye
V	**Trigeminal** (3 branches- Opthalmic, maxillary and mandibular)	Pons	Temperature, touch and pain to areas served	Chewing
VI	**Abducens**	Pons	Proprioception of eye	Lateral movement of eye
VII	**Facial**	Pons	Proprioception of face	Facial expression. Secretion of saliva and tears
VIII	**Auditory**	Inner ear	Vestibular - balance Cochlear - hearing	None
IX	**Glossophary -ngeal**	Medulla	Maintenance of B.P. (Sensory from carotid sinus)	Secretion of saliva from parotid gland
X	**Vagus**	Medulla	Sensation from viscera. Parasympathetic innervation of G.I. tract	Visceral muscle movement
XI	**Accessory**	Medulla and C1 - C5	Proprioception of areas supplied. Movement of head	Swallowing
XII	**Hypoglossal**	Medulla	Proprioception of tongue	Movement of tongue

Oh! Oh! Oh! To Touch And Feel A Green Vegetable, Ah! Heaven!

The Respiratory System

Anatomy

The Physiology of Ventilation

Nervous & Chemical Control

Gas Transport

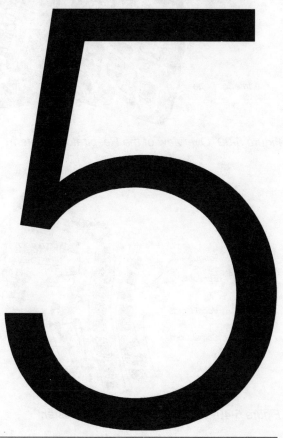

Basic Anatomy

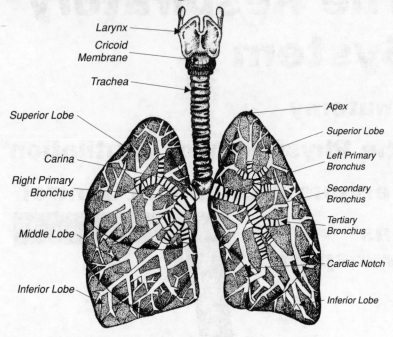

Figure 5-39 Overview of the Respiratory System

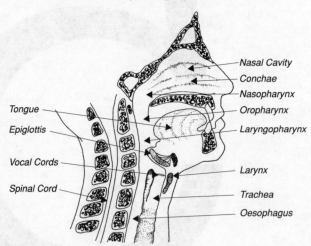

Figure 5-40 The Upper Respiratory System

The Nose

The external portion of the nose is composed of cartilage overlaid with skin and is lined internally with mucous membrane. The openings to the exterior are called the external nares. The mucous membrane, together with the nasal hairs, trap dust and dirt that is drawn into the nose during respiration. The nasal cavity is divided by the nasal septum. The internal portion communicates with the paranasal sinuses and the nasopharynx through the internal nares.

The interior portion of the cavity is called the vestibule. The walls of the vestibule are lined with mucous membrane in the same way as the external nasal cavity. In addition, the walls are deeply ridged, known as the nasal conchæ. These conchæ take the form of folds of membrane, following the form of the turbinate bones. The conchæ warm and moisten the air before it is drawn into the lungs. In the roof of the vestibule are the olfactory bulbs, which are nerve endings of the olfactory nerve, which provides the sense of smell.

The nose warms, moistens and filters air, is the organ of smell and forms a resonating chamber for the modification of speech sounds.

The Pharynx

The pharynx is a muscular tube lined with mucous membrane. It is divided into three parts; the nasopharynx, the oropharynx and the laryngopharynx.

The nasopharynx extends from immediately posterior to the nasal cavity to the level of the soft palate. The nasopharynx communicates with both the nose and the inner ear. The openings from the nose are the internal nares of the nasal cavity. The openings into the inner ear, via the eustachian tubes, are concerned with the equalisation of air pressure to the inner part of the eardrum. In the rear wall of the nasopharynx are the pharyngeal tonsils, or adenoids, which are a collection of lymphatic tissue. The walls are lined with ciliated epithelium, the cilia of which transports the mucus from the nose towards the oropharynx. The oropharynx is situated at the rear of the oral cavity and extends from the soft palate to the level of the hyoid bone, (at the top of the larynx). The walls are lined with stratified squamous epithelium. The palatine tonsils lie at the rear of the oropharynx, either side of the opening into the oral cavity. The lingual tonsils lie at the base of the tongue. The oropharynx is a passageway for both food and air.

The laryngopharynx extends from the level of the hyoid bone and divides at its lower end into the oesophagus and the trachea. It is lined with stratified squamous epithelium.

The Larynx

The larynx is the passageway that connects the pharynx with the trachea. It is comprised of nine cartilages:

The Epiglottis   The Thyroid Cartilage   The Cricoid Cartilage
The Arytenoid Cartilages (2)   The Corniculate Cartilages (2)
The Cunieform Cartilages (2)

During swallowing, the larynx as a whole moves upward, meeting the free underside of the epiglottis. This closes off the larynx and prevents the passage of food into the airway.

The epiglottis is a large leaf-shaped cartilage that is attached anteriorly to the thyroid cartilage. The posterior portion is free to move.

The thyroid cartilage is formed from two fused pieces of cartilage and forms the anterior wall of the larynx. It can be felt on the outside of the neck as the Adams Apple.

The cricoid cartilage is an 'O' shaped, complete ring of cartilage. It forms the whole of the posterior wall of the larynx and part of the anterior wall. Between the thyroid cartilage and the cricoid cartilage is the crico-thyroid membrane, the site of emergency cricothyroidostomy.

The arytenoid, corniculate and cunieform cartilages are interconnected cartilages which form the method of controlling the vocal cords, producing and modifying speech and other sounds.

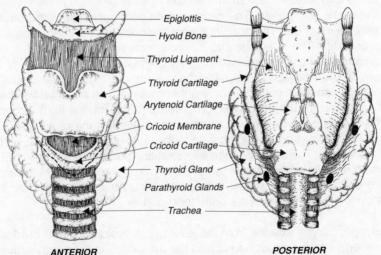

Epiglottis
Hyoid Bone
Thyroid Ligament
Thyroid Cartilage
Arytenoid Cartilage
Cricoid Membrane
Cricoid Cartilage
Thyroid Gland
Parathyroid Glands
Trachea

ANTERIOR   **POSTERIOR**

Figure 5-41 The Larynx

The Trachea

The trachea extends from the larynx to the primary bronchi. It is immediately anterior to the oesophagus and is composed of between 16 and 20 'C' shaped, incomplete, cartilage rings, (with the open part of the C at the rear) and with smooth muscle between the rings. The open ends of the rings are joined at the rear by smooth muscle and elastic connective tissue, which serves to allow for slight expansion of the oesophagus when swallowing, and to retain the shape and patency of the airway when not swallowing. It is lined with pseudostratified epithelium, with goblet and ciliated cells, which provide and waft mucus upwards to be eventually swallowed, so protecting the airway against dust particles. The trachea bifurcates at about the level of the fifth thoracic vertebra into the left and right primary bronchi. At this point is a small ridge of cartilage, the carina, which is the part of the respiratory system which is most sensitive to dust or other foreign objects and is the centre for the cough reflex.

The Lungs

The lungs are a pair of organs in the thoracic cavity. They are enclosed in the pleural membranes, the outer of which is the parietal pleura and the inner of which is the visceral pleura. Between the pleura is a potential space, the pleural cavity, which is filled with serous fluid, which lubricates the two surfaces of the pleura as they slide over one another during respiration. Without this lubrication, the pleura would rub together and cause intense pain (plueritic rub) on breathing.

The right lung comprises three lobes, divided by fissures. The left lung comprises two lobes, divided by one fissure. The left lung has a depression, the cardiac notch, which accommodates the heart.

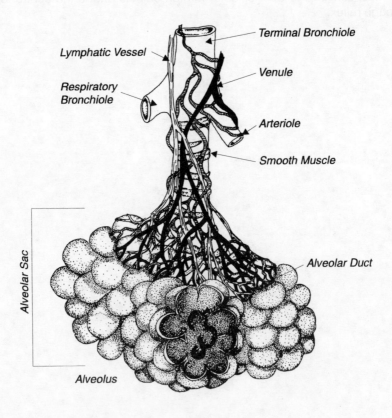

Figure 5-42 A Lobule of the Lung

The Bronchi

The complete bronchial tree consists of the trachea, primary bronchi, secondary bronchi, tertiary bronchi, bronchioles, terminal bronchioles and respiratory bronchioles. The bronchi are composed of complete rings of cartilage interspersed with smooth muscle and lined with pseudostratified ciliated epithelium, for the same reasons as the trachea and pharynx. The further down the bronchial tree, the less cartilage and the more smooth muscle is found.

The primary or left and right main bronchi serve one lung each. They are the widest part of the respiratory system below the trachea. The right primary bronchus is wider, more vertical and shorter than the left, making it the prime candidate for obstruction by foreign objects such as inhaled peanuts etc. The secondary bronchi are also known as lobar bronchi as they serve the two lobes, or sections, of the left lung and the three lobes of the right lung. The tertiary or segmental bronchi each serve a segment of each lobe. The terminal bronchioles serve a lobule each.

A lobule is a bag of connective tissue which contains an arteriole, a venule, a lymphatic vessel and a terminal bronchiole. The terminal bronchioles branch within the lobule to form respiratory bronchioles which each serve an individual alveolar sac. Gas exchange takes place across the alveolar-capillary membranes.

The Physiology of Ventilation

Pulmonary ventilation consists of inspiration and expiration. The pulmonary cycle consists of inspiration, expiration, pause. The pause is necessary for the chemical changes taking place as a result of the ventilation to have an effect on the nervous system. The movement of air into and out of the lungs depends on pressure changes, governed partly by Boyles Law, which states that the volume of a gas changes inversely with pressure, assuming the temperature is constant. Inspiration occurs when intrathoracic pressure falls below atmospheric pressure. Contraction, and therefore flattening, of the diaphragm and contraction, and therefore shortening, of the external intercostal muscles increases the size of the thorax, thus decreasing the intrapleural pressure so that the lungs expand. Expansion of the lungs decreases intrapulmonic pressure so that the air moves down the pressure gradient into the lungs.

Expiration occurs when intrapulmonic pressure is higher than atmospheric pressure. Relaxation of the diaphragm and the external intercostals results in elastic recoil of the chest wall and lungs, which increases intrapleural pressure, lung volume decreases and intrapulmonic pressure increases so that air moves down the pressure gradient out to the atmosphere.

Forced inspiration involves the accessory muscles, (sternocleidomastoids, scalenes and pectoralis minor). Forced expiration involves contraction of the internal intercostals and abdominal muscles.

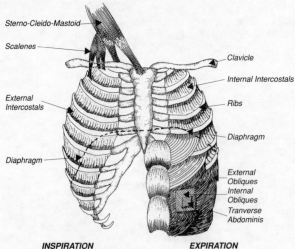

INSPIRATION   EXPIRATION

Figure 5-43 The Respiratory Muscles

Volumes and Capacities

During normal, quiet breathing, approximately 500ml of air is moved into and out of the respiratory system. However, only about 350ml of this air takes place in gas exchange, because there is a 150ml dead air space, in the pharynx, trachea and bronchi. This dead air space is increased with any equipment that forms part of a closed system, such as endotracheal tubes. A catheter mount can add as much as 50ml to the dead air space, which means that 550ml of air has to be moved into and out of the system for 350ml to reach the alveoli. This increases the effort required for respiration.

If the body requires more oxygen due to, for instance, greater exertion, the lungs can be expanded to a greater degree by the use of accessory muscles. This provides an additional inspiratory reserve volume of approximately 3100ml of air. When added to the normal tidal volume, this gives an inspiratory capacity of 3600ml.

If additional air needs to be moved out of the lungs, for instance for coughing or blowing, there is an expiratory reserve volume of about 1200ml.

If the lungs are emptied as much as possible and are then inflated as much as possible, this gives a total air movement of approximately (3100 + 500 + 1200) = 4800ml, which is known as the vital capacity.

There is always some air left in the lungs following expiration, otherwise the lungs would collapse. This volume is approximately 1200ml. When added to the vital capacity, this gives a total lung capacity of approximately 6000ml.

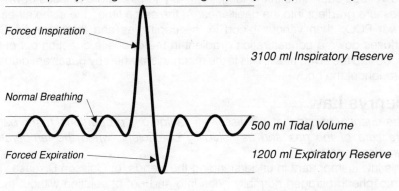

Figure 5-44 Respiratory Volumes

Some Laws of Physics

Boyles Law

The pressure of gas in a closed container is inversely proportional to the volume of the container, provided the temperature is constant.

This means that when the volume of the thoracic cavity is increased, as in inspiration, the pressure of the gas in the thoracic cavity is reduced, creating a pressure gradient, which forces air in from the atmosphere. (Providing the trachea is open.) The opposite happens for expiration.

Charles Law

The volume of a gas is directly proportional to its' absolute temperature, if the pressure remains constant.

As gases enter the respiratory passages and lungs, they are warmed, providing an increase in volume. This reduces the amount of work required from the muscles, making breathing physically easier.

Daltons Law

Each gas in a mixture of gases exerts its' own pressure, as if the other gases were not present.

This pressure is known as partial pressure, denoted as "P". The partial pressure of a gas in a mixture can be determined by multiplying the percentage content of the gas by the total pressure. Normal atmospheric air has 21% oxygen and a pressure of 760 mmHg. The partial pressure of oxygen (PO_2) in atmospheric air is calculated as follows: $PO_2 = 21\% \times 760 = 159.6$ (160 mmHg). Inspired air has a higher partial pressure of oxygen (PO_2) than the venous capillaries in the lungs. The oxygen therefore diffuses down the pressure gradient into the capillaries. At the same time, the same air has a lower PCO_2 than venous blood in the capillaries and therefore the CO_2 diffuses down a concentration gradient in the opposite direction out of the blood into the alveolar air. This is the mechanism whereby gases are diffused throughout the body.

Henrys Law

The quantity of gas that will dissolve in a liquid is proportional to the partial pressure of the gas and its solubility coefficient, when the temperature remains constant.

This law is important in understanding the Bends, or Caisson Disease. The atmospheric nitrogen normally goes into and out of solution without much being used in the body. (It is thought to play some part in protein synthesis in the cells) When the atmospheric pressure rises, as in diving, the amount of nitrogen dissolved increases. When the pressure is suddenly reduced, as in surfacing too quickly, the gas cannot dissolve out and diffuse into the atmospheric air quickly enough and nitrogen bubbles are formed. The incidence of bubbles can be reduced by either surfacing slowly or going into a decompression chamber, where the pressure is gradually reduced.

The effects of Henrys Law are also used in hyperbaric oxygenation, where anaerobic bacteria, (which cannot live in the presence of free oxygen) are killed by raising the pressure of oxygen in atmospheric air, thereby increasing the partial pressure, creating a greater concentration gradient with the blood, which causes the PO_2 to be raised in the blood.

Control Mechanisms

In normal, healthy people, the basic drive for respiration is high levels of carbon dioxide in the blood. The basic rhythm of respiration is controlled by portions of the central nervous system in the medulla and pons. These are the medullary rhythmicity centre (consisting of the inspiratory area and the expiratory area), the pneumotaxic area and the apneuistic area.

The nervous impulses that drive these areas come from the chemoreceptors in the aortic and carotid bodies. The basic rhythm can be modified by cortical influences, the inflation reflex, changes in body temperature, pain, stretching the anal sphincter and irritation of the respiratory mucosa.

In the normal resting state, inspiration lasts for about two seconds and expiration lasts about three seconds. At the end of expiration, the inspiratory area is inactive, but after three seconds it spontaneously becomes active, possibly by the same process that makes the SA node in the heart spontaneously active. (Intrinsic excitability), and also responds to impulses from various receptors (see below). The impulses from the inspiratory area last for about two seconds and travel to the muscles of inspiration via various nerves. After two seconds the inspiratory area becomes inactive again and expiration occurs passively. There is then a pause, whilst the CO_2 in the blood builds up and the inspiratory area becomes active again. Therefore, inspiration is the result of chemical changes in the blood and also the self excitation of the inspiratory area, whilst expiration is passive. Inspiration can be increased and expiration made an active process by the use of accessory muscles of respiration.

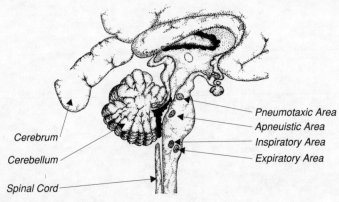

Cerebrum
Cerebellum
Spinal Cord

Pneumotaxic Area
Apneuistic Area
Inspiratory Area
Expiratory Area

Figure 5-45 Respiratory Centres

When the chemoreceptors in the carotid and aortic bodies and the chemosensitive area in the medulla are subjected to high acidity levels (low pH), due to high levels of CO_2 (see later) they stimulate the inspiratory area. This sends a signal down the spinal cord to the nerves controlling the diaphragm and the external intercostal muscles, causing them to contract. This forces air into the lungs. The lungs have stretch receptors in them that are stimulated when a certain pressure is reached (the inflation or Hering-Bruer reflex). This sends a signal back (positive feedback) to inhibit the inspiratory area and thereby initiate expiration (a passive process).

The normal arterial PCO_2 is 40mmHg. If there is even a small rise, (hypercapnia), the chemosensitive area in the medulla and the chemoreceptors in the aortic and carotid bodies are stimulated. These cause the inspiratory area to become highly active.

The pneumotaxic area normally inhibits the inspiratory area, which effectively limits inspiration before the lungs become too full. The apneuistic area sends stimulatory impulses to the inspiratory area that activate it and prolong inspiration, thus inhibiting expiration. This occurs when the pneumotaxic area is inactive. When the pneumotaxic area is active, it overrides the apneuistic area to extend the time of inspiration and bring the accessory muscles of inspiration into play, (the sternocleidomastoid, the pectoralis major and scalenes) thereby increasing the amount of air taken in. The highly active inspiratory area also activates the normally inactive expiratory area. This sends impulses to the abdominal muscles and the external intercostals to forcibly decrease the capacity of the thoracic cavity and achieve forced expiration. This allows the lungs to be ventilated at a higher cyclical rate.

The oxygen chemoreceptors are only sensitive to large decreases in PO_2. If the PO_2 falls from the normal 105mmHg to around 70mmHg, the oxygen chemoreceptors become stimulated and send impulses to the inspiratory area. However, should the arterial PO_2 fall much below 70mmHg, the cells of the inspiratory area suffer from hypoxia and do not respond well to any stimulation from any source. Persons who are used to a high PCO_2, such as chronic bronchitics and asthmatics, use the oxygen chemoreceptors (hypoxic drive) to stimulate respiration.

The respiratory area has connections with the cortex and cerebellum, which allows a person to voluntarily alter their pattern of breathing, such as for speaking. However, when the PCO_2 reaches a certain low level, the inspiratory area is stimulated, forcing an inspiration.

Gas Transport

Oxygen

3% of the oxygen transported in the blood is dissolved in the plasma and 97% is carried on the heme portion of the haemoglobin (which consists of 4 atoms of Fe), as oxyhæmoglobin.

As PO_2 rises, the amount of oxygen in association with the hæmoglobin is increased until saturation is reached. When PO_2 reaches approximately 105 mmHg, the hæmoglobin is fully saturated. As PO_2 falls, the percentage saturation also falls. This saturation is the measurement used in pulse oximetry. Red blood cells change colour as they become saturated with oxygen and this change is used to determine the percentage of oxygen saturation.

The blood will pick up a nearly a full load of oxygen from the lungs even when the PO_2 is as low as 60 mmHg. However, when the PO_2 reaches about 40 mmHg, the hæmoglobin saturation is down to 75% and at 10 mmHg, the saturation falls dramatically to 13%. Tissues that are using large amounts of oxygen, such as muscles, induce a low PO_2 in the blood, thereby forcing the hæmoglobin to give up its oxygen to the tissues.

Hæmoglobin also gives up its oxygen in conditions of low pH, (high acidity). This condition is brought about by metabolism, where CO_2 is released from tissues. Therefore, where there is high tissue activity, with consequent low pH, the need for oxygen will be high. This need is satisfied more easily because the oxygen will split from the hæmoglobin more easily.

Highly active cells also give off heat, which is another factor that will cause oxygen to split more readily from hæmoglobin.

Carbon Dioxide

7% of the carbon dioxide carried in the blood is directly dissolved in the plasma. 23% is combined with the globin portion of hæmoglobin as carbaminohæmoglobin. 70% is carried as bicarbonate ion (HCO_3^-) This transport is as a result of the following reaction, which goes either way according to the conditions:- $CO_2 + H_2O < > H_2CO_3 < > H^+ + HCO_3^-$

This means that H_2CO_3 (Carbonic Acid) will dissociate in carbon dioxide and water or, alternatively, hydrogen ions and bicarbonate ions.

As CO_2 diffuses into tissue capillaries and enters the red blood cells, it reacts with H_2O in the presence of carbonic anhydrase, to form H_2CO_3.

The H_2CO_3 dissociates into H^+ ions and HCO_3^- ions. The H^+ ions combine mainly with Hb. The HCO_3^- ions leave the red blood cells and enter the plasma. In exchange, Cl^- ions diffuse from plasma into the red blood cells. This exchange of negative ions maintains the ionic balance between red blood cells and plasma and is known as the chloride shift. The Cl^- ions that enter the red blood cells combine with K^+ ions to form KCl. The HCO_3^- ions that enter the plasma combine with Na^+ ions (the main ion in extracellular fluid) to form $NaHCO_3$. The net effect of all these reactions is that CO_2 is carried from tissue cells as bicarbonate ions in plasma

Deoxygenated blood returning to the lungs contains CO_2 dissolved in plasma, CO_2 combined with globin as carbaminohæmoglobin and CO_2 incorporated in HCO_3^- ions. The reverse of the above takes place

Just as an increase in CO_2 (and therefore lower pH) in blood causes O_2 to split more easily from Hb, the binding of O_2 to Hb causes the release of CO_2 from the blood. In the presence of O_2, less CO_2 binds in the blood. This reaction, called the Haldane effect, occurs because when O_2 combines with Hb, the Hb becomes more acidic. Also, the more acidic Hb releases more H^+ ions that bind to HCO_3^- ions to form H_2CO_3. The H_2CO_3 breaks down into $H_2O + CO_2$, and the CO_2 is released from the blood into the alveoli. In tissue capillaries, blood picks up more CO_2 as O_2 is removed from Hb. In pulmonary capillaries, blood releases more CO_2 as O_2 is picked up by Hb.

The amount of CO_2 transported in blood is significantly influenced by PO_2. As CO_2 leaves the tissue cells and enters blood cells, it causes more O_2 to dissociate from Hb, (the Bohr effect) and thus more CO_2 combines with haemoglobin and more HCO_3^- ions are produced. As O_2 passes from alveoli into blood cells, Hb becomes saturated with O_2 and becomes a stronger acid. The more acidic Hb releases more H^+ ions which bind to HCO_3^- ions to form H_2CO_3. The H_2CO_3 dissociates into $H_2O + CO_2$ and the CO_2 is released from the blood into the alveoli.

The Heart

Anatomy & Physiology

The Coronary Circulation

Extrinsic & Intrinsic Control

The Electrical Conduction System

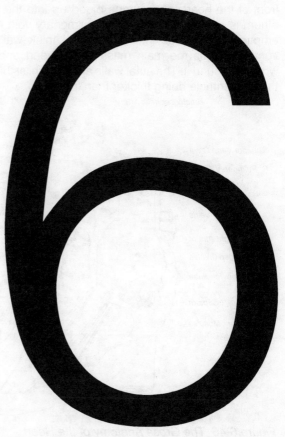

Gross Anatomy

The heart is the size of its owners clenched fist. It lies posterior to the sternum and costal cartilages in the mediastinum a mass of tissue between the lungs. It rests on the central part of the diaphragm anterior to the oesophagus. The whole heart is invaginated in the pericardial cavity a fibrous bag lined with a serous membrane which permits the heart free movement whilst contracting. The walls of the heart are made up of branching fibres of cardiac muscle.

The heart has four chambers, two atria or collecting chambers and two ventricles or pumping chambers. (Both types pump). The arrangement of the chambers is not simple. The right atrium which is really an enlargement of the superior and inferior vena cavae lies along the right border of the heart and opens on its left side into the triangular right ventricle. This lies on the front of the heart and pumps blood up into the pulmonary artery. The left atrium is roughly square with a pulmonary vein entering at each corner. It empties downwards into the conical thick walled left ventricle. The left ventricle forms the main mass of the heart and the other chambers are wrapped round it. The atrial walls are thin whilst the ventricular walls are thick the left ventricle being thicker than the right.

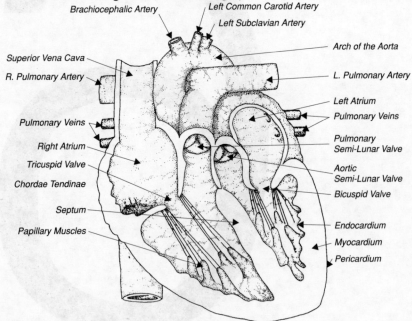

Figure 6-46 The Gross Anatomy of the Heart

Structure of the heart wall

The heart wall consists of three layers. The outer layer (the pericardium), the middle layer (the myocardium), and the inner layer (the endocardium).

The pericardium is a thin serous membrane covering the myocardium and is the visceral layer of the double coated pericardial sac. This sac keeps the heart in place in the mediastinum whilst allowing the heart to change shape as it beats. Between the two layers is a potential space called the pericardial cavity which is filled with serous fluid to provide lubrication as the heart moves. The middle layer of the heart is the myocardium which is the muscular part of the heart. The myocardium is made up of involuntary striated branched muscle fibres which are arranged in interlacing bundles. (see diagram) The inner layer is the endocardium which is a thin layer of epithelium on a basement membrane of connective tissue.

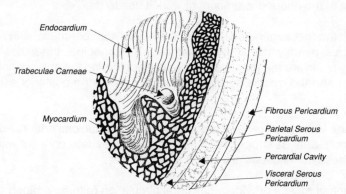

Figure 6-47 The Heart Wall

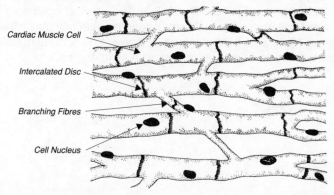

Figure 6-48 Cardiac Muscle

Blood Supply to the Heart

The left coronary artery arises from the ascending aorta, runs under the left atrium and divides into the anterior interventricular and circumflex branches. The anterior interventricular branch follows the anterior interventricular sulcus (a groove in the surface of the heart) and supplies oxygenated blood to both ventricles. The circumflex branch supplies oxygenated blood to the walls of the left ventricle and left atrium.

The right coronary artery also originates as a branch of the ascending aorta. It runs under the right atrium and divides into the posterior interventricular and marginal branches. The posterior interventricular branch follows the posterior interventricular sulcus and supplies the walls of both ventricles with oxygenated blood. The marginal branch transports oxygenated blood to the wall of the right ventricle. The left ventricle receives the largest blood supply because of the enormous amount of work it has to do.

Most of the deoxygenated blood drains into the coronary sinus which discharges directly into the right atrium. The principal tributaries of the coronary sinus are the great cardiac vein which drains the anterior aspect of the heart and the middle cardiac vein which drains the posterior aspect of the heart.

Most parts of the body receive branches from more than one artery and where two or more arteries supply the same region they usually connect with each other. These connections are called anastomoses.

These anastomoses provide a collateral circulation (alternate blood supply) for blood to reach a particular organ or tissue. When a major coronary artery is about 90% obstructed blood will flow through the collateral vessels. Although most collaterals are quite small heart muscle can stay alive as long as as little as 10-15% of normal supply is present. This does not mean that the muscle will not be damaged or complain as in angina.

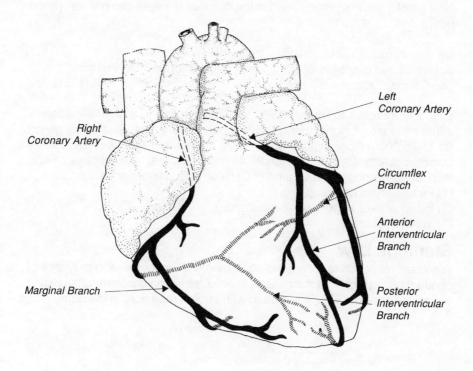

Figure 6-49 The Coronary Blood Supply

Cardiac Output

Cardiac output is the amount of blood pumped into the aorta in one minute (minute volume). It is equal to the amount of blood pumped out with each beat (stroke volume) multiplied by the number of beats per minute. (heart rate).

Cardiac output = stroke volume x heart rate.
Stroke volume averages of 70ml. Heart rate averages of 70-75 bpm.
So:- Cardiac Output = SV x HR = 70 x 72 = approx. 5,000ml (AT REST)

This may increase to up to 20,000 ml with exercise in a normal person, a 400% increase. A highly trained athlete may have a reserve of 600% giving up to 30,000 ml per minute during very strenuous exercise. This reserve output is greatly affected by ischaemic heart disease, valvular disease and myocardial damage. The volume of Cardiac output is dependent on :-
(1) Frequency of heart rate,
(2) Blood pressure (peripheral resistance),
(3) Venous return.

Starlings Law

The heart responds to increased stretching with an increase in the force of contractions. It therefore matches cardiac output with venous return avoiding distension of veins. This is achieved with stretch receptors in the atria.

Blood Flow through the Heart

Deoxygenated blood from the body tissues enters the right atrium from the superior and inferior vena cavae. 70% of the blood falls, due to gravity, through the tricuspid valve into the right ventricle and the atrial systole completes the emptying of the atrium. At the same time oxygenated blood from the lungs enters the left atrium via the four pulmonary veins and once again 70% falls through the bicuspid valve into the left ventricle. The left atrium contracts forcing the rest through.

The contraction of the left ventricle forces the bicuspid valve closed and blood is pumped through the semi-lunar aortic valve into the aorta to the body. The contraction of the right ventricle forces the tricuspid valve closed and blood is pumped through the semi-lunar pulmonary artery valves into the pulmonary artery to the lungs.

The systole of the ventricles snaps the tricuspid and bicuspid valves closed giving the first heart sound (LUB). At the end of the ventricular contraction the semi-lunar aortic and pulmonary artery valves snap closed due to back pressure which gives the second heart sound (DUPP). The atria take time to fill again and this causes the pause after the lub dupp.

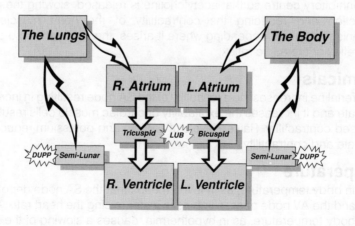

Figure 6-50 Blood Flow through the Heart

Extrinsic Control of the Heart

The autonomic nervous system acts as an accelerator and brake, both at the same time. Any change in one allows the other to take over or be suppressed. Several factors can make the changes.

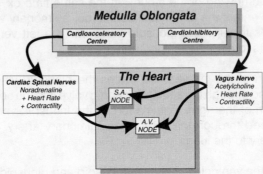

Figure 6-51 Nervous Control of the Heart

Baroreceptors

These are situated in the carotid sinus of the carotid artery, the aorta (near the junction with the pulmonary artery) and in the right atrium. They are stretch receptors. When they are stretched they send a message to the cardioinhibitory centre so that acetylcholine is released, slowing the rate of contraction and reducing the contractility of the heart muscle. The mechanism is called, depending where it arises, the atrial reflex the carotid sinus reflex or the aortic reflex.

Chemicals

Noradrenaline increases the excitability of the SA node resulting in increased heart rate and it increases the excitability of cardiac muscle cells resulting in increased contractility. Raised levels of sodium and potassium reduces the heart rate and contractility.

Temperature

A rise in body temperature, as in fever, means that the SA node depolarises faster and the AV node passes impulses faster raising the heart rate. A drop in the body temperature, as in hypothermia, causes a slowing of the rate of discharge of the SA node and a slowing of the rate of transfer at the AV node resulting in a reduction in heart rate and the muscle cells are less excitable, resulting in less contractility.

Emotion

Excitement leads the brain to release more adrenaline causing an increase in heart rate and contractility. Depression and tragedy result in the release of acetylcholine resulting in a decrease in heart rate and contractility.

Sex

Females tend to have a higher pulse rate than males.

Age

The rate tends to change with age. The average adult is 60 - 80 but from birth (140) this tends to slow until the average adult rate is reached for some decades and then in old age it tends to slow down more and become more erratic.

Baroreceptors	**Chemicals**	**Temperature**
Carotid Sinus reflex *Aortic reflex* *Right Atrial reflex* *= -bpm & -contractility*	*Noradrenaline = -bpm* *Acetylcholine = -bpm* *+K = -bpm & - Contractility* *+Na = -bpm & -Contractility* *+Ca = +bpm & +Contractility*	*+°C = +bpm & +Contractility* *-°C = -bpm & -Contractility*

The Electrical Conduction System of the Heart

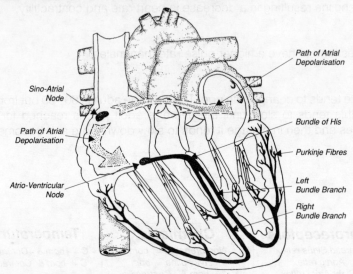

Figure 6-52 The Electrical Conduction System

The heart is innervated by the autonomic nervous system but this only alters the rate that the sino-atrial node depolarises. The heart rate is controlled primarily by the rate of self-depolarisation of the sino-atrial node.

The cell membrane is leaky in that the membrane is very permeable to the passage of sodium (Na^+) ions even in the resting state. As a result the sodium ions diffuse through the sodium channels into the cell causing the membrane potential to change to a more positive value. (The difference is in the region of 70mv). This process is called depolarisation.

Once the membrane potential reaches its threshold level an action potential is generated. As the action potential develops the membrane becomes less permeable to Na^+ ions and more permeable to potassium (K^+) ions. As K^+ ions diffuse out of the cell through the potassium channels the inside of the cells become more negative. This is repolarisation. This reversal of charge stops the action potential. Through the operation of the sodium and potassium pumps Na^+ ions are actively transported out of the cells and K^+ ions are actively transported into the cells. Then the influx of Na^+ ions initiates another action potential and the process of self-excitation repeats itself again and again.

As the sino-atrial node depolarises the action potential that it generates is transmitted along conduction fibres to depolarise the atria in such a manner that the muscular wall contracts forcing the blood downwards into the ventricles. The wave of depolarisation is transmitted from muscle fibre to muscle fibre which achieves a wave of contraction. The individual muscle fibres are connected by intercalated discs which allow the transmission of the depolarisation from fibre to fibre.

As the wave of depolarisation reaches the atrioventricular node there is a pause and then the action potential is transmitted down a tract of conducting fibres, the Bundle of His, to be distributed to the ventricular muscle fibres. The actual contraction is stimulated by the Purkinje fibres that emerge from the bundle branches and innervate the myocardium.

The depolarisation of the atria produces the P wave which is followed by a pause as the wave is delayed by the atrioventricular node. The Q wave is the first negative (downward) deflection before a positive (upward) deflection. The R wave is the first positive deflection whether or not there is a Q wave. The S wave is a downward deflection following an R wave. The QRS complex as a whole records the passage of the wave down the Bundle of His and into the myocardium. The T wave records the repolarisation of the ventricles. There is a pause after the QRS complex which is the time taken for the sodium and potassium channels to open and the voltages to reverse. The repolarisation of the atria is hidden as it occurs during the QRS complex, which is much stronger.

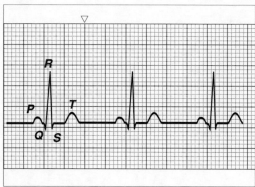

Figure 6-53 Normal Sinus Rhythm

Each small square on the ECG = 0.04 sec. Each Large square = 0.20 sec. Normal values are :- P-R interval = 0.12 - 0.20 sec. QRS = 0.08 - 0.12 sec. S-T segment = 0.27 - 0.33 sec. The whole cardiac cycle normally last about 0.8 seconds. (60 seconds divided by 75 beats per minute).

Blood Vessels & Blood

Veins & Arteries

Fluid Dynamics

Blood Pressure

Blood

The Lymphatic System

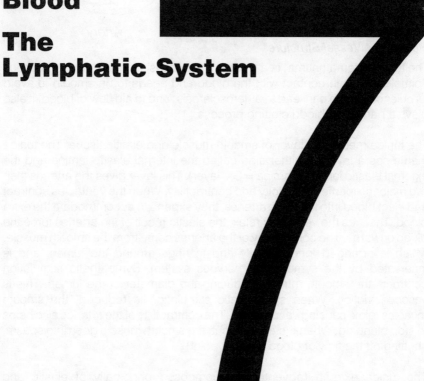

The Structure of Veins and Arteries

Arteries have three main layers. The inside layer is the tunica intima, the middle layer is the tunica media and the outer layer is the tunica adventitia.

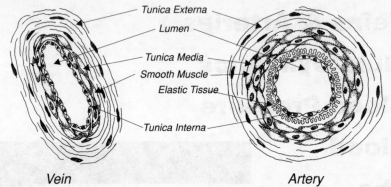

Vein   Artery

Figure 7-54 Vessel Structure

The tunica interna (intima) is a smooth lining, consisting of simple squamous epithelium. It is in contact with the blood and needs to be smooth to avoid turbulence (which can lead to atherosclerosis) and to aid flow of blood. It also plays a part in the blood clotting process.

The tunica media is a layer of smooth muscle and elastic tissue. The tunica media has a layer on either side called the internal elastic lamina and the external elastic lamina. (lamina = Gk. layer). This layer gives the arteries their two major properties, elasticity and contractility. When the ventricles contract and eject blood into the large arteries, they expand to accommodate the extra blood. Then, as the ventricles relax, the elastic recoil of the arteries force the blood onwards. The contractility of the arteries come from the smooth muscle, which is arranged longitudinally and in rings around the lumen. and is innervated by the sympathetic nervous system. Sympathetic stimulation contracts the smooth muscle, reducing the diameter of the lumen. This is vasoconstriction. When sympathetic stimulation is reduced, the smooth muscles relax, causing vasodilation. The contractility of the arteries also helps to stop bleeding. When the artery is cut, the smooth muscle goes into spasm, shutting off the flow of blood (up to a point).

The tunica externa (adventitia) is composed principally of elastic and collagenous fibres. and serves to hold the artery in place in the body, maintain its shape, (especially under the pressure of systole), and provide protection.

Arterioles

Arterioles are very small, almost microscopic arteries that deliver blood to the capillaries. As they become more distal to the arteries and more proximal to the capillaries, they have less elastic tissue and more smooth muscle than arteries, thus enabling the autonomic nervous system to significantly adjust blood pressure, or to maintain falling blood pressure in the early stages of shock.

Metarterioles are microscopic vessels that connect arterioles and venules, as a thoroughfare channel, with capillaries leading from them. A small amount of gas exchange is achieved from the metarterioles, but the bulk is carried out from the capillaries.

Capillaries

Capillaries are microscopic vessels that connect arterioles to venules. They are found near to virtually every cell in the body. The distribution of capillaries varies with the activity of the tissue. The epidermis, the cornea and lens of the eye and cartilage have no capillary network.

The primary function of capillaries is to facilitate the exchange of gases, wastes, nutrients and water between the blood and the tissues.

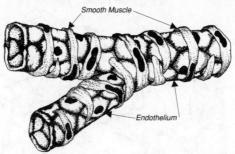

Smooth Muscle

Endothelium

Figure 7-55 A Capillary

The structure of the capillary wall, a one cell thick layer of endothelium, allows the easy passage of substances, with only one cell thickness to pass through. The wall of the capillary allows the passage of substances by four routes, depending on the type and location of the capillary. These routes are: Through the cell membrane directly by diffusion, as in most muscle tissue; through the endothelial junctions; via pinocytic vesicles; and through fenestrations (windows). Some fenestrations are completely open, as in the kidneys, and some are closed by a thin membrane, such as in the villi of the small intestine, the choroid plexuses of the ventricles of the brain, the ciliary processes of the eye and the endocrine glands.

Blood flow through capillaries is controlled by the action of smooth muscles around the arterioles, metarterioles and by the precapillary sphincters. The centre for control is the vasomotor centre in the medulla, with connections from the aortic and carotid baroreceptors. This control is vital to the maintenance of systemic blood pressure. If the flow of blood through the capillary bed is restricted, this diverts blood flow directly from the arterioles to the venules, along the thoroughfare channel s, cutting out a large capacity of blood vessels, so increasing the volume of blood in the systemic circulation. The diameter of the arterioles and metarterioles can also be reduced, thereby increasing peripheral resistance, thereby increasing systemic blood pressure.

Venules and veins are of a similar construction to arteries and arterioles except that they have thinner walls, and do not have the internal and external elastic laminae. The long veins, especially in the legs, contain valves to prevent the backflow of blood, which assists venous return.

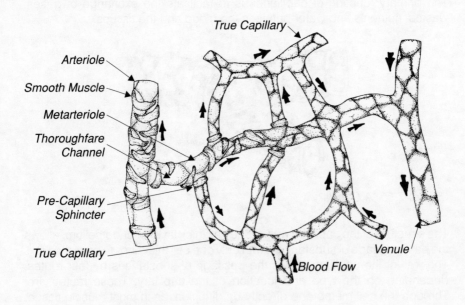

Figure 7-56 Capillary Blood Flow

Anastomoses

Most parts of the body receive branches from more than one artery. In such areas the distal ends of the vessels unite. The junction of two or more vessels supplying the same body part is called an anastomosis. They may also occur between the origins of veins and between arterioles and venules. Anastomoses between arteries provide alternate routes by which blood can reach an organ or tissue. Thus, if a vessel is occluded by disease, injury or surgery, circulation to the part of the body is not necessarily stopped. The alternate route of blood to a body part through an anastomosis is known as collateral circulation. An alternate blood supply can also come from non-anastomosing vessels that supply the same region of the body. Arteries that do not anastomose are known as end arteries. Occlusion of an end artery interrupts the blood supply to the whole segment of tissue, causing ischaemia and eventually necrosis of the tissue. (Infarction)

Blood and Interstitial Fluid

The velocity of blood flow is slowest in the capillary network. This allows the exchange of gases, water nutrients and wastes between the capillary blood and the interstitial fluid to take place. The exchanges take place down pressure gradients.

There is a net pressure gradient of 8mm Hg from the arterial capillary blood to the interstitial fluid and -7mm Hg from the venous capillary blood to the interstitial fluid. (In effect a 7mm Hg pressure gradient from the interstitial fluid to the blood) These pressures are the net result of several opposing forces, due to the blood 'and interstitial fluid pressure (hydrostatic pressure) and the osmotic pull of the proteins and ions in the blood and interstitial fluid, (osmotic pressure).

The arterial blood has a hydrostatic pressure (BHP) of about 30mm Hg and an osmotic pressure (pull) (BOP) of about 28mm Hg. The interstitial fluid has a hydrostatic pressure (IFHP) of about 0mm Hg and an osmotic pressure (pull) (IFOP) of about 6m m Hg. At the venous end of the capillary bed, the blood hydrostatic pressure (BHP) is about 15mm Hg and the blood osmotic pressure (pull) (BOP) of about 28mm Hg. The interstitial fluid has a hydrostatic pressure (IFHP) of 0mm Hg and an osmotic pressure (pull) (IFOP) of about 6mm Hg. The lymph capillaries have a hydrostatic pressure of -1mm Hg (they drain the interstitial space, taking excess fluid, proteins and bacteria etc.)

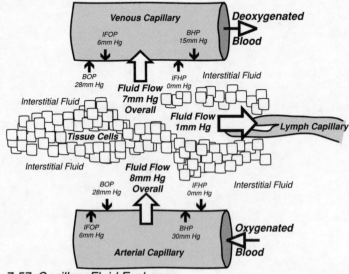

Figure 7-57 Capillary Fluid Exchange

Blood Pressure

Blood pressure is the pressure exerted on the wall of the blood vessel by the blood. In clinical use, the pressure in the arteries is usually measured, although the central venous pressure (CVP) is also used. Blood pressure is determined by cardiac output and peripheral resistance. Blood flows through the closed system of blood vessels due to the different blood pressures in the various parts of the cardiovascular system. Blood flow is directly proportional to blood pressure. Blood always flows fro m regions of high blood pressure to regions of low blood pressure (down the pressure gradient) and pressure differences are related to cardiac output and peripheral resistance. This results in the blood passing through arteries at high speed but through capillaries at low speed, allowing for the exchange of gases and nutrients.

The mean pressure in the aorta is 100 mmHg. Since the heart pumps in a pulsating manner, the systemic arterial pressure in a resting young adult fluctuates between 120 mmHg (systolic) and 80 mmHg (diastolic). As blood leaves the left ventricle and flows through the systemic circulation, its pressure falls progressively t o 0 mmHg by the time it reaches the right atrium. Resistance in the aorta is nearly 0 but it is close to the powerfully contracting left ventricle, so pressure is high. (100 mmHg). Likewise, resistance in the large arteries is also quite low, but since these are close to the aorta, the mean arterial pressure is still high (about 95-97 mmHg). In small arteries, resistance increases rapidly and pressure decreases rapidly to about 85 mmHg at the beginning of the arterioles.

Resistance in arterioles is the highest in the cardiovascular system, accounting for about one half of the total resistance to blood flow. Pressure decreases in arterioles from 85 to about 30 mmHg. As blood next passes into the arteriole end of a capillary, its pressure is about 30 mmHg and at the venous end of the capillary, the pressure is about 10 mmHg. The decrease in pressure in the venous system is not as abrupt as in the arterial system. The pressure at the beginning of the venous system, t hat is in the venules, is about 10 mmHg. The pressure continues to decrease in veins and the venae cavae to about 0 mmHg in the right atrium. A great deal of the resistance in veins is caused by their compression from surrounding tissues and pressure in the abdomen.

The Autonomic Nervous System

Blood pressure can be affected in several ways, using the autonomic nervous system. Baroreceptors in the aortic and carotid bodies send impulses to the vasomotor centre in the medulla, which continuously maintains a state of moderate vasoconstriction. Increases or decreases in vasomotor tone cause a raising or lowering of blood pressure by several means.

Cardiac output

The amount of blood ejected into the aorta per minute. This is the main determinant of blood pressure. The cardioacceleratory and cardioinhibitory centres adjust the rate and contractility of the heart.

Blood reservoirs

The systemic blood volume can be increased by increasing the vasomotor tone and squeezing blood from reservoirs such as in the spleen, liver, large abdominal veins and the vessels of the skin.

Peripheral resistance

The vasomotor centre causes vasoconstriction, which raises the peripheral resistance and diverts blood from the capillary bed, which directly raises blood pressure. Resistance is also related to blood viscosity, blood vessel length and blood vessel radius.

Blood viscosity (thickness) is increased by dehydration, polycythaemia or severe burns, which increase blood pressure by raising the blood osmotic pressure and pulling water into the intravascular space (the blood vessels). A depletion of plasma proteins or red blood cells as a result of haemorrhage or anaemia decreases blood viscosity and therefore pressure, by lowering the blood osmotic pressure, which becomes lower than the interstitial fluid osmotic pressure, pulling water into the interstitial space. This is normally countered by vasoconstriction.

Resistance is directly proportional to blood vessel length, the longer the vessel, the greater the resistance. Vasoconstriction reduces the length of the vessels by cutting out the capillaries, thereby lowering resistance. Resistance is inversely proportional to the fourth power of the radius of the blood vessel. (e.g. If the radius of the blood vessel is reduced by one half, the resistance is increased by sixteen times). If the reduced radius involves many arterioles, the overall peripheral resistance is greatly increased.

All these effects are balanced and adjusted by changing the diameter of different blood vessels at different places in the body, in order to achieve the desired effect.

Chemicals

Adrenaline and noradrenaline increase the rate and contractility of the heart. They cause vasoconstriction of abdominal and cutaneous arterioles and veins but vasodilation of cardiac and skeletal muscle arterioles. Histamine is a powerful vasodilator.

Blood

Blood has three functions:

1. Transport of oxygen from the lungs to the cells of the body; carbon dioxide from the cells to the lungs; nutrients from the gastrointestinal tract to the cells; waste products from cells; hormones from the endocrine system to the cells; heat from various cells.

2. Regulation of pH through buffers; normal body temperature through the heat-absorbing and cooling properties of its water content; the water content of cells principally through dissolved sodium ions (Na+) and proteins.

3. Protection against blood loss through the clotting mechanism; foreign microbes and toxins through certain white blood cells that are phagocytic or specialised proteins such as antibodies, interferon and complement.

Blood has two components:

1. Formed elements (cells and cell-like structures) 45% of blood volume.
2. Plasma (a liquid containing dissolved substances) 55% of blood volume.

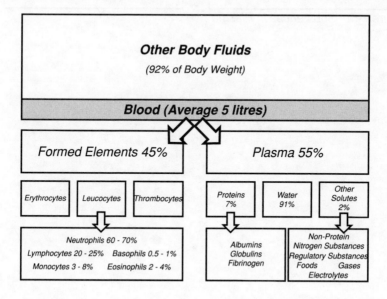

Figure 7-58 The Formed Elements of Blood

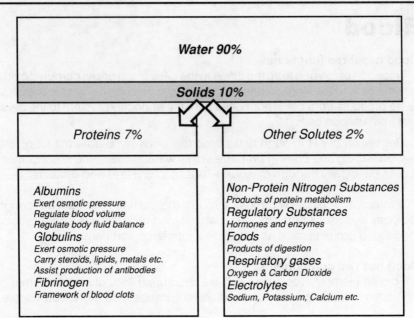

Figure 7-59 Substances in Plasma

Prevention of blood loss

Blood loss is prevented through three main mechanisms.
1. Vascular spasm
2. Platelet plug formation
3. Coagulation

1. Vascular spasm

When a blood vessel other than a capillary is damaged, the circularly arranged smooth muscle in its wall contracts immediately. Such a vascular spasm reduces blood loss for several minutes to several hours, during which time the other mechanisms can go into operation. The spasm is probably caused by the damage to the smooth muscle and from reflexes initiated by pain receptors.

2. Platelet plug formation

Platelets are normally disc-shaped. Under the surface of the cell membrane are tube-like structures composed of myosin and actin. In the cytoplasm are several substances that are actively involved in stemming blood loss. platelet-derived growth factor (PDGF) causes vascular endothelial cells, vascular smooth muscle cells and fibroblasts to proliferate in order to help repair the damaged blood vessel wall. ADP, ATP and serotonin are enzyme systems which produce fibrin stabilising factor which helps to strengthen a blood clot.

In the first phase of platelet plug formation, platelets come into contact with the damaged blood vessel wall. The platelets adhere to the damaged collagen. When they adhere, the platelets undergo a change in shape and nature. The platelet become s irregularly shaped and forms numerous projections which connect with other platelets. The platelets also secrete the stored blood coagulation factors. Serotonin and thromboxane function as vasoconstrictors, which help reduce the blood flow locally. ADP al so makes other platelets that arrive on the scene sticky, which makes them adhere to the rapidly forming platelet plug. The platelet plug is initially loose, but the arrival of coagulation factors in the extrinsic and intrinsic pathways tightens the plug by the formation of fibrin threads.

3. Coagulation

Normally, blood maintains its liquid state as long as it remains in an undamaged vessel. If it is in contact with the air it forms a gel. Eventually, the gel separates into a solid and liquid. The liquid is serum, which is plasma with the coagulation factors removed. The coagulation factors have been removed by the solid to form a clot.

Coagulation is a complex process in which the activated form of one coagulation factor catalyses the activation of the next factor in the sequence. Once the process is initiated, there is a cascade of events that results in the formation of large quantities of product. For purposes of discussion, the clotting mechanism is described as a sequence of three basic stages:
1. Formation of prothrombin activator
2. Conversion of prothrombin into thrombin by prothrombin activator.
3. Conversion of soluble fibrinogen into insoluble fibrin by thrombin.

Prothrombin activator formation is initiated by the interplay of two mechanisms, the extrinsic and the intrinsic pathways of blood clotting.

The extrinsic pathway is so-called because it involves substances which are produced by cells outside the blood. Cells throughout the body, but particularly in the brain, lungs and intestines have a protein called thromboplastin (tissue factor) on their surface. When tissue is damaged, tissue factor combines with blood factors and Ca^{2+} ions, in a chain, to form prothrombin activator.

The intrinsic pathway is more complex and is so-called because it is initiated by tissue factor from damaged cells that line the damaged blood vessel itself, and from factors within the blood itself. In the intrinsic pathway, factors also activate other factors, (in the presence of phospholipids from damaged platelets and Ca^{2+} ions) to form new factors which lead to the formation of prothrombin activator. The diagram shows the two pathways in detail, but it must be remembered that these pathways only lead to the formation of prothrombin activator, which is in itself only a step on the complete coagulation process.

Completion of coagulation

Prothrombin is activated to form thrombin, which in the presence of Ca^{2+} activates fibrinogen to form loose fibrin threads. Thrombin, in the presence of factor XIII converts loose fibrin threads into stabilised fibrin threads, which hold the platelets firmly together and stabilise the clot. The clot then retracts by the action of the fibrin threads pulling the platelets together, which pulls the sides of the wound together, further reducing haemorrhage.

Thrombin has a positive feedback effect, the more that is produced, the more the acceleration of the production of prothrombin activator. Platelet phospholipids are also produced by adhering platelets, causing more platelets to adhere, accelerating the clot growth. These accelerants are prevented from forming a massive clot by blood flow washing away coagulation factors except from within the platelet plug.

Formed clots contain inactive plasminogen which is activated by blood factors to plasmin, which dissolves fibrin threads to break up the clot when the tissue is repaired. The clot material is then absorbed.

Blood groups

There are at least 300 blood group systems that can classify blood. The two major systems that concern us are the ABO system and the Rh system.

The ABO system

Erythrocytes have antigens on their surface, called agglutinogens, classified as A or B, Type A blood has type A agglutinogens, group B blood has type B agglutinogens, group AB blood has both A and B, and group O blood has neither A nor B.

Plasma has antibodies called agglutinins. These 'are part of the bodies defence system against foreign material and the agglutinins will attack specific agglutinogens on the surface of foreign erythrocytes. Agglutinin a will attack agglutinogen A and agglutinin b will attack agglutinogen B. Group A blood has agglutinin b, group B blood has agglutinin a, group AB blood has neither a nor b, group O blood has both a and b.

If a person with blood group A receives a transfusion of blood group B, the agglutinin b in the type A blood will attack the agglutinogen B on the foreign erythrocytes, causing erythrocyte clumping and destruction of the foreign blood. A person with blood group B receiving blood group A will similarly attack the foreign blood with their agglutinin b. However, a person of blood group AB, having no agglutinins to attack foreign blood with and is therefore able to receive blood from any blood group. Any person can receive blood group O as there are no agglutinogens to attack. This system is summarised in the diagrams below.

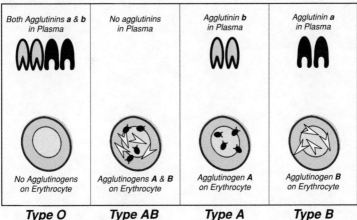

Both Agglutinins **a** & **b** in Plasma	No agglutinins in Plasma	Agglutinin **b** in Plasma	Agglutinin **a** in Plasma
No Agglutinogens on Erythrocyte	Agglutinogens **A** & **B** on Erythrocyte	Agglutinogen **A** on Erythrocyte	Agglutinogen **B** on Erythrocyte
Type O	**Type AB**	**Type A**	**Type B**

Figure 7-60 The ABO System

The Rh system

This system is of interest with pregnancy. If a man is Rh positive (has Rh agglutinogens on erythrocytes) and he fathers a child in a Rh negative mother, (Rh factor being a dominant gene, the foetus will be Rh positive) the mother will then develop anti-Rh agglutinins due to the presence of the Rh factor on the foetal erythrocytes. If he then fathers a second child in the same mother, the mothers anti-Rh agglutinin will attack the foetal blood. There are two avenues to approach the problem. The mother can be immunised with anti-Rh gamma$_2$globulin before the second pregnancy, to tie up the anti-Rh agglutinins, or, if this is not done, the foetal blood can be changed for Rh negative blood, which will not be attacked. If the mother is Rh positive, there will be no problem as there will be no anti-Rh agglutinins. The Rh and other blood type factors cause haemolytic disease of the newborn (Erythroblastosis fetalis).

The Lymphatic System and Immunity

The lymphatic system consists of a fluid called lymph, vessels that transport lymph called lymphatic vessels (lymphatics), and a number of structures and organs that contain lymphatic (lymphoid) tissue.

Essentially, lymphatic tissue is a specialised form of reticular connective tissue that contains large numbers of lymphocytes. Lymphatic tissue occurs in the body in various ways. Lymphatic tissue not enclosed in a capsule is referred to as diffuse lymphatic tissue. This is the simplest form of lymphatic tissue and is found in the connective tissue of mucous membranes of the gastrointestinal tract, respiratory passageways, the urinary tract and reproductive tract. Lymphatic nodules also do not have capsules and are oval shaped concentrations of lymphatic tissue. Most lymphatic nodules are solitary small and discrete. Such nodules are found in the lamina propria of the mucous membranes of the gastrointestinal tract, the respiratory tract, the urinary tract and the reproductive tract. Some lymphatic nodules occur in multiple large aggregations in specific parts of the body. Among these are the tonsils, follicles in the small intestine and the appendix. Lymphatic organs of the body - the lymph nodes, spleen and thymus gland - all contain lymphatic tissue enclosed by a connective tissue capsule. Bone marrow also produces lymphocytes, so is also considered a component of the lymphatic system.

Lymphatic vessels originate as microscopic vessels in spaces between cells called lymph capillaries. Lymph capillaries may occur singly or in extensive plexuses. They originate throughout the body, except in avascular tissue, the central nervous system, splenic pulp and bone marrow. Lymph capillaries also differ from blood capillaries in that they end blindly. Blood capillaries have an arterial and venous end. In addition, lymph capillaries are structurally adapted to ensure the return of proteins to the cardiovascular system when they leak out of blood capillaries.

Close examination of lymph capillaries reveals that there are minute openings between endothelial cells making up the capillary wall that permit fluid flow easily into the capillary, but prevent the flow of fluid out of the capillary, much like a one-way valve would operate. Note also that the outer surface of the endothelial cells of the capillary wall are attached to the surrounding tissue by structures called anchoring filaments. During oedema, there is an excessive accumulation of fluid in the tissue, causing tissue swelling. This swelling produces a pull on the anchoring filaments, making the openings between cells even larger so that more fluid can flow into the lymph capillary.

Just as blood capillaries converge to form venules and veins, lymph capillaries unite to form larger and larger lymph vessels, called lymphatic vessels. Lymphatic vessels resemble veins in structure but have thinner walls and more valves and contain lymph nodes at various intervals along their length. Lymphatic vessels of the skin travel in loose subcutaneous tissue and generally follow veins. Lymphatic vessels of the viscera generally follow arteries, forming plexuses around them. Ultimately, lymphatic vessels deliver their lymph into two main channels - the thoracic duct and the right lymphatic duct.

When plasma is filtered by blood capillaries, it passes into the interstitial spaces; it is then known as interstitial fluid. Fluid movement between blood capillaries and body cells depends on hydrostatic and osmotic pressures. When this fluid passes from interstitial spaces into lymph capillaries, it is called lymph (lympha Gk=clear water). Lymph from lymph capillaries is then passed to lymphatic vessels that run toward lymph nodes. At the nodes, afferent vessels penetrate the capsules at numerous points and the lymph passes through the sinuses of the nodes. Efferent vessels from the nodes either run with afferent vessels into another node of the same group or pass on to another group of nodes. From the most proximal group of each chain of nodes, the efferent vessels unite to form lymph trunks. The principal trunks are the lumbar, intestinal, bronchomediastinal, subclavian and jugular trunks.

The principal trunks pass their lymph into two main channels, the thoracic duct and the right lymphatic duct. These two ducts then discharge the lymph into the cardiovascular system at the junction of the subclavian vein and the internal jugular vein on the left and right sides respectively.

The flow of lymph from tissue spaces to the large lymphatic ducts to the subclavian veins is maintained primarily by the milking action of skeletal muscles. Skeletal muscle contractions compress lymphatic vessels and force lymph towards the subclavian veins. Lymphatic vessels, like veins, contain valves, and the valves ensure the movement of lymph towards the subclavian veins. Respiratory movements also helps with lymph flow. These movements create a pressure gradient between the two ends of the lymphatic system. Lymph flows from the abdominal region, where the pressure is higher, toward the thoracic region, where it is lower.

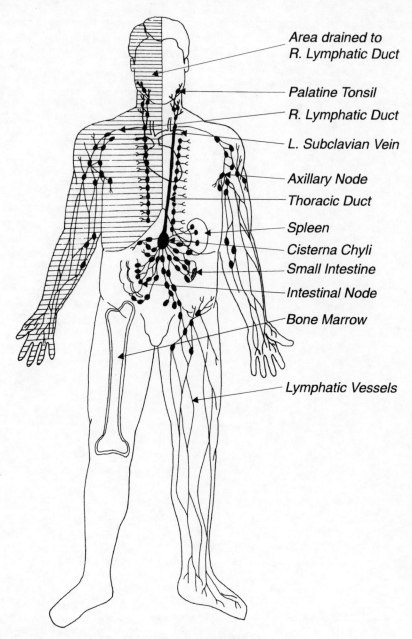

Area drained to
R. Lymphatic Duct

Palatine Tonsil

R. Lymphatic Duct

L. Subclavian Vein

Axillary Node

Thoracic Duct

Spleen

Cisterna Chyli

Small Intestine

Intestinal Node

Bone Marrow

Lymphatic Vessels

Figure 7-61 Overview of the Lymphatic System

Study Guide

Reading Material

Study Techniques

Subjects To Be Studied

The Entry Test

Weekly Study Programme

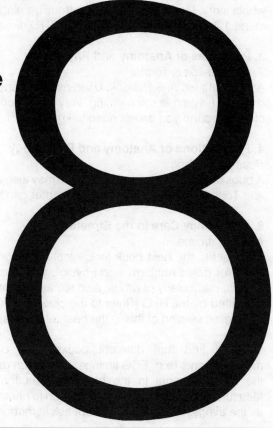

Suggested Reading Material

(Apart from this book)

1.Ambulance Service Basic Training(Green Book)
NHSTD.
A back up for anatomy and physiology, also basic techniques of clinical management. Lots of basic facts (recently updated). Available from Training Schools and the NHSTD direct.

2. Extended Training in Ambulance Aid (Blue book)
NHSTD
Mainly specific techniques of clinical management, but also A. & P. facts to learn. Don't forget that they are called background notes, as they are not the whole story. Usually available free from Training Schools just before starting stage 1, but can be obtained from NHSTD direct.

3. Principles of Anatomy and Physiology
Anagnostakos & Tortora
A very detailed A. & P. book. Used as a reference book when Ross & Wilson does not fully explain something. Very deep, containing many details and lots of background you do not need to know, which may confuse you.

4. Foundations of Anatomy and Physiology
Ross and Wilson
A book of reference for A. & P. but you may also want to look in Anagnostakos and Tortora for full detail. A whole chapter can be read.

5. Emergency Care in the Streets
Nancy Caroline
At present , the best book for clinical conditions and management. Not so good for basic Anatomy and Physiology. Watch out for Americanisation of names, particularly of drugs, also techniques of management which are not permitted by the NHS (Refer to the blue book for these). I will be producing an English version of this in the near future. Watch this space.

You will find that different books have different values for various measurements (e.g. ECG timings, respiration rates, blood volumes etc) Use the measurements in the blue book as the course is based on this. Measurements are variable from person to person. There ain't no such animal as the average person. If in doubt ask somebody.

The place to start is the normal anatomy and physiology of the various systems of the body. Begin with the basic functions of one system at a time, ignoring everything else. Then look at the structure (anatomy) of that system then look at how it works (physiology). Once you have studied the basic system anatomy and physiology then look at its control mechanisms (what makes it work). After looking at each system in isolation you can study the inter-relationships between systems and from there the whole maintenance of the body (homeostasis).

For the anatomy and physiology component of your study, the main book will be Anagnostakos & Tortora, with back-up from Ross & Wilson for another view if you don't understand. Use A. & T. as a reference book as it is very deep and complex in most places. The study guides at the end of the chapters will be useful to see if you have understood the subject. Try to answer the questions. If you can't, go back to Ross & Wilson and re-read it then refer to A. & T. and then try to answer the question again, preferably in writing for exam practice.

For the clinical conditions the best book is Emergency Care in the Streets, as Nancy Caroline has a good style of writing, which is almost conversational. She takes you through the conditions step by step, explaining what is happening with each one.

Study techniques

In order to gain the maximum out of your reading you must organise your study time properly. Try to arrange a quiet space and time so that you are able to devote your full attention to studying.

Try to spend one to two hour blocks in study. Less than one hour and you will spend more time preparing than working and unless you are experienced at study techniques you will find it hard to concentrate for more than two hours at once. Try to organise regular study periods so that learning becomes part of your regular routine. Try to have everything you need for study together before you begin - pens paper books etc. It is very disturbing to your concentration to break off to find a pen.

If something completely baffles you and you can't find the answer in a book, write the question down (otherwise you will forget) and ask somebody who is likely to know.

Learning aids

Audio tapes
Dictate reading material on to audio tape. This helps in several ways:
a) Making the tape is an intensive study exercise.
b) Listening to the tape will require concentrated attention.
c) You can replay the tape as often as you wish.
d) You can listen to the tape while doing routine tasks.
e) You can use the tapes to write notes or questions from.

Notes
Try to use key words notes instead of traditional longhand notes. Traditional notes are notoriously boring to write and you are less likely to read them once written. You must be careful to use words phrases and mnemonics to stimulate your memory. Then use the notes to write questions (and answer them!)

Books
Only read intensively those parts of books that you need to. You will retain more information if you read selectively than by cramming indiscriminately. If you don't understand something in one book refer to another. If still in doubt ask somebody.

SQ3R

This is a method of reading effectively. It means:-

Survey Question Read Review Recite.

With practice this technique will help you to get more out of your reading. Most people do not utilise their reading skills efficiently and consequently waste time and energy. ''

Survey

This means scan the reading task, read headings, summarise first and last sentences (or paragraphs). THEN:

Question

Set yourself questions: Do I need to read all this? What do I know already? (Beware of assuming you know the subject well enough. Try the questions at the end of the chapter if you think you know it.) What do I want from this material? How can I best obtain it? You may need to write yourself questions to aid your reading. THEN:

Read

Actually read the text (or parts of it) as a result of the questions above. THEN

Review

This is the time to rehearse or revise. Practice what you have learnt, set yourself questions. Go back and re-learn the parts that you fail on. THEN

Recite

Tell somebody else. You must do this to be sure that
a) you have learnt
b) You can remember
c) you are correct
d) You can fill in gaps.

Initially this method of reading may seem to be time consuming and difficult but with practice it will enable you to carry out reading tasks more efficiently and also retain more.

Subjects to be studied

These are the subjects which make up stage one of the NHSTD Extended Training course. Stage one consists mainly of revision of anatomy and physiology knowledge that has been pre-learnt for the course, with fuller explanations and therefore fuller understanding. You need to know this much to take stage one. Stage two consists mainly of clinical conditions and you need the anatomy and physiology knowledge to fully understand the conditions. However do not go into the clinical conditions too much before you know the anatomy and physiology.

Part 1   Cells tissues and cavities of the body
a) The basic structure of the cell.
b) The basic functions/properties of a cell
c) The chromosomes and their ability to transfer genetic material
d) The different types of tissue and where they are to be found.
e) The properties of cardiac skeletal & smooth muscles and the basic chemistry of contraction.
f) The types and names of bones with special reference to the skull and maxillo-facial bones.
g) Types of joints.
h)The main muscles of the body especially of respiration.
i)Identify the systems regions and cavities of the body and locate the organs within each

Part 2   Chemical reactions within the body
a) Electrolytes - what are they?
b) The structure of atoms (very briefly)
c) Positive and negative ions.
d) The acid-base balance of the body.
e) How the body maintains the normal pH balance
f) Body fluids.
g)Diffusion and osmosis.

Part 3The Endocrine System
a) The function of the pituitary gland
b) The thyroid and parathyroid gland
c) The adrenal glands with emphasis on the bodily effects that aldosterone, adrenaline and noradrenaline have.
d) The islets of Langherhan

Part 4   The Nervous System
a) The structure and types of nerve cells.
b) The structure and functions of the brain. (Functions in brief except for the medulla.)

c) The sensory (afferent) and motor (efferent) nerves and pathways.
d) The spinal cord and its nerve pathways.
e)The function and distribution of cerebro-spinal fluid.
f) All the cranial nerves (including functions)
g) The autonomic nervous system with emphasis on the sympathetic and the parasympathetic effects.
h) The nerve reflexes (1. Spinal 2. Cortical 3. Co-ordinating 4. Autonomic)

Part 5 The Respiratory system
a) Respiratory organs: Nasal cavity, Pharynx, Larynx, Trachea, Bronchi and bronchioles, Alveoli and lungs
b) The muscles of respiration and their nerves.
c) The cycle of respiration.
d) Internal and external respiration.
e) The nervous and chemical control of respiration.
f) The interchange of gases and their partial pressures.
g) Lung capacities: 'Complemental air, Tidal volume, Supplemental volume, Residual air etc

Part 6 The Heart
a) The structure of the heart and it's blood supply.
b) The flow of blood through the heart and its control.
c) The electrical conduction system and its nervous control.
d) The chemo/baro receptors and their effects on the heart and vessels.
e) The cardiac cycle.
f) Cardiac output and its control by: Heart rate, Contractility, Starlings law, Elasticity and recoil of blood vessels.
g) Heart sounds.

Part 7 Blood and its vessels
a) The structure of veins and arteries.
b) Diffusion and osmosis in relation to nutrient and waste transport.
c) The effect of the autonomic nervous system on blood vessels.
d) The maintenance of normal blood pressure.
e) The pulse and factors affecting it.
f) The main arteries and veins.
g) The lymphatic system.
h) The composition of blood.
i) Erythrocytes and thrombocytes.
j) Types of leucocytes and their function (briefly)
k) The process of blood clotting (Extrinsic and intrinsic pathways).
l) Blood groups and cross-matching.
m) The immune process.

The Entry Test

Assuming that you are eligible to take the entry test for the full NHSTD Extended Training Course, (which means that you have to be a full-time employee of the NHS Ambulance Service, qualified to Ambulance Technician grade with at least 12 months post qualification experience on A & E work), you can take the entry test at any time that it is available and as many times as you like (or can stand!)

The entry test consists of three parts.

1. Multiple choice / true or false questions. (30 of each)
In the multiple choice questions believe me there is only one completely correct answer. If it seems to be ambiguous, you have probably misread it. Choose the answer that is most correct from the choices. You cannot say "it depends". In the true or false questions read the question carefully as they are sometimes phrased in the negative.

Go through the paper and answer the questions you are sure about. Then count up and see if you have enough to pass. If you have answered 51 or 52 questions and you are completely sure they are right you can stop there. You do not need to answer all the questions to pass. You need 85% to pass which means 51 correct out of 60. If you have answered less than 51 that you are sure about, this is not enough and you must go over the paper again to see if there are any more that you can answer. After this, only make intelligent guesses to the best of your ability.

2. Short answer questions.
These are reasonably simple in operation if you go about them in a structured way. First of all read all the questions and make sure you know what they want. Then decide which order you want to answer them. It is easiest to start with the ones you know the most about as you will get a lift from being able to answer them and you may gain some time to answer the difficult ones.

The easiest way to start each question is to revert to the key words method as used in note taking. List some key words or headings in the top corner of the paper (the examiner may even take these into account if you run out of time as they show you are on the right track). Then list them out on the answer paper and leave some lines in between. Then all you have to do is fill in the gaps. This way if you run out of inspiration, the headings will remind you and they will also assist you in answering the question in a logical sequence. If you are reasonable at drawing include a diagram if you have time.

However if it says list then do so, as this is all that is required. Any further explanation will probably not attract any marks as you have not answered the question in the way that they asked. It also wastes time.Talking of time there are five questions to be answered in one and a half hours. This does not work out at 18 minutes per question as you will need time to read all the questions first and also to read your answers over at the end to look for stupid mistakes. Allow fifteen minutes at the most for writing each answer and stick rigidly to it. If you go over time on one question leave it and come back to it if you have time.

3. Practical tests.
These consist of:
1. Resuscitation. Failure to achieve 100% competence in this test nullifies all other elements of the examination.

2. Examination and diagnosis of an unconscious patient.

3. Management of a trauma patient If you can't do these by this stage of your career you may as well not start at all.

You will also have to undertake a personal interview, the panel consisting of at least one member of the Local Ambulance Advisory Panel, usually a physician, anaesthetist or senior nurse and an Ambulance Service Trainer. The interview panel will take into account the entry examination results, applicants attitude, sense of responsibility, motivation and personal records.

10 Week Study Programme

Week 1

Section 1 Cells tissues and cavities of the body
a) The basic structure of the cell.
b) The basic functions/properties of a cell
c) The chromosomes and their ability to transfer genetic material (very briefly)

d)The different types of tissue and where they are to be found.
e) The properties of cardiac skeletal and smooth muscles and the basic chemistry of their contraction.

Week 2

Section 1 Cells tissues and cavities of the body
 f) The types and names of bones with special reference to the skull and maxillo-facial bones.
g) The main muscles of the body especially of respiration.
h) Identify the systems regions and cavities of the body and locate the organs within each.

Week 3

Section 2 Chemical reactions within the body
a) Electrolytes - what are they?
b) The structure of atoms (very briefly)
c) Positive and negative ions.
d) The acid-base balance of the body.
e) How the body maintains the normal pH balance
f) Body fluids.
g) Diffusion and osmosis.

Section 3 The Endocrine System
a)The function of the pituitary gland
b)The thyroid and parathyroid gland
c)The adrenal glands with emphasis on the effects of aldosterone, adrenaline and noradrenaliine
d)The islets of Langherhan

Week 4

Section 4 The Nervous System
a) The structure and types of nerve cells.
b) The structure and functions of the brain. (Functions in brief except for the medulla.)
c) The sensory (afferent) and motor (efferent) nerves and pathways.
d) The spinal cord and its nerve pathways.
e) The function and distribution of cerebro-spinal fluid.

Week 5

Section 4 The Nervous System

f) All the cranial nerves (functions)

g) The autonomic nervous system with emphasis on the sympathetic and the parasympathetic effects on the body.

h) The nerve reflexes (1. Spinal 2. Cortical 3. Co-ordinating 4. Autonomic)

Week 6

Section 5 The Respiratory system

a)Respiratory organs:Nasal cavity Pharynx Larynx Trachea Bronchi and bronchioles Alveoli and lungs

b) The muscles of respiration and their nerves.

c) The cycle of respiration.

d) Internal and external respiration.

Week 7

Section 5 The Respiratory system

e) The nervous and chemical control of respiration.

f) The interchange of gases and their partial pressures.

g) Lung capacities Complemental air Tidal volume Supplemental volume Residual air etc

Week 8

Section 6 The Heart

a) The structure of the heart and it's blood supply.

b) The flow of blood through the heart and its control.

c) The electrical conduction system and its nervous control.

Week 9

Section 6 The Heart

d) The chemo/baro receptors and their effects on the heart and vessels.

e) The cardiac cycle.

f) Cardiac output and its control by: Heart rate, Contractility, Frank Starlings law, Elasticity and the recoil of blood vessels.

g) Heart sounds.

Week 10

Section 7 Blood and its vessels

a) The structure of veins and arteries.

b) Diffusion and osmosis in transportation of nutrients and waste.

c) The effect of the autonomic nervous system on blood vessels.

d) The maintenance of normal blood pressure.

e) The pulse and factors affecting it.

f) The main arteries and veins.

g) The lymphatic system.

h) The composition of blood and blood clotting.

Glossary

Definitions of terms

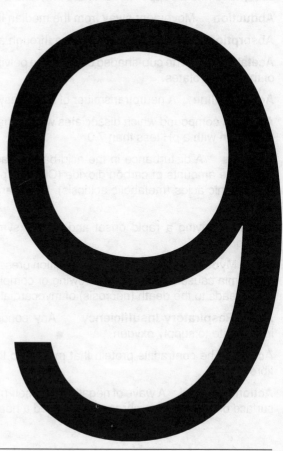

This glossary is intended to provide brief definitions of terms used in the text. You need to understand what all these words mean.

A   An abbreviation meaning without, as in Apnoea.

Abdomen   The large cavity below the diaphragm and above the pelvis. Contains the stomach, spleen, liver, gallbladder, pancreas, small intestine and most of the large intestine.

Abdominal   Relating to the abdomen.

Abdominopelvic   Inferior compartment of the ventral body cavity that is subdivided into an upper abdominal cavity and a lower pelvic cavity.

Abduction   Movement away from the median line of the body.

Absorption   Passage of a substance through a membrane.

Acetabulum   The cup-shaped cavity in the pelvis in which the rounded head of the femur rotates.

Acetylcholine   A neurotransmitter of the parasympathetic nervous system.

Acid   A compound which dissociates with formation of hydrogen ions (H+). A solution with a pH less than 7.0.

Acidosis   A disturbance in the acid-base balance of the body caused by excessive amounts of carbon dioxide (CO_2) respiratory acidosis) or of lactic and organic acids (metabolic acidosis). It is characterised by a a pH of less than 7.35.

Acute   Having a rapid onset and severe symptoms and being of short duration.

Acute Myocardial Infarction   A condition present when a period of cardiac ischaemia caused by sudden narrowing or complete occlusion of a coronary artery leads to the death (necrosis) of myocardial tissue.

Acute Respiratory Insufficiency   Any condition in which breathing is inadequate to supply oxygen

Actin   The contractile protein that makes up thin myofilaments in muscle fibre.

Action Potential   A wave of negativity that self-propogates along the outside surface of a neuron membrane. Also called a nerve impulse.

Active Transport   The movement of substances, usually ions, across cell membranes against a concentration gradient requiring the expenditure of energy.

Adduction   Movement towards the median line of the body.

Adenoids   The pharyngeal tonsils.

Adrenaline   The hormone produced by the adrenal glands, with alpha and beta stimulating properties.

Adrenal Cortex   The outer portion of the adrenal gland.

Agglutinin   A specific principle or antibody in blood serum, capable of causing the clumping of bacteria, blood corpuscles or particles.

Agglutinogen   A genetically determined antigen located on the surface of erythrocytes. Basis for the ABO and Rh systems of blood classification.

Agonal   Pertaining to the period of dying.

Air Embolism   An air bubble introduced into the bloodstream.

Air Hunger   Another term for acute dyspnoea, or shortness of breath with rapid, laboured breathing.

Albumin   The most abundant (60%) and smallest of the plasma proteins, which functions primarily to regulate the osmotic pressure of plasma.

Aldosterone   A mineralocorticoid produced by the adrenal cortex, that affects the rate of sodium and water reabsorption and potassium excretion.

Alkaline   In chemistry, having a pH greater than 7.0 (In physiological, terms having a pH greater than 7.35).

Alkalosis   An abnormal condition of acid-base balance that results when the body loses too much carbon dioxide by hyperventilation, (respiratory alkalosis) or too much acid from, for example vomiting, (metabolic alkalosis). It may also be caused b y excessive intake of alkaline substances such as antacids or sodium bicarbonate. The latter especially when sodium bicarbonate is given during cardiopulmonary resuscitation.

All-or-none   In muscle physiology, muscle fibres of a motor unit contract to their fullest extent or not at all. In neuron physiology, if a stimulus is strong enough to initiate an action potential an impulse is transmitted along the entire neuron at a constant and minimum strength.

Alpha (a) receptor   A centre located in the walls of small arteries and veins, that when stimulated by alpha (sympathetic) drugs or hormones, causes the vessel to constrict.

Alveolar duct   Branch of a respiratory bronchiole around which alveoli and alveolar sacs are arranged.

Amino acid   An organic acid that is the basic unit from which proteins are formed.

Aminophylline   A drug used to relax smooth muscle in bronchioles.

Amplitude   Height, usually of an ECG wave or complex.

Ampoule   A sealed glass container of medication.

Anabolism   Synthetic energy-requiring reaction whereby small molecules are built into large ones.

Anaerobic   Not requiring molecular oxygen. (as in bacteria).

Analgesia   Absence of normal sense of pain.

Anaphase   The third stage of mitosis in which the chromatids that have separated at the centromeres have moved to opposite poles.

Anaphylaxis   A hypersensitivity (allergic) reaction in which IgE antibodies attach mast cells and basophils causing them to produce mediators of anaphylaxis (histamine and prostaglandins) that bring about increased blood permeability increased smooth muscle contraction and increased mucus production. Examples are hay fever, bronchial asthma and anaphylactic shock.

Anaemia   Condition of the blood in which the number of functional red blood cells or their haemoglobin content is reduced.

Aneurysm   A sac-like enlargement of a blood vessel caused by a weakening of its wall.

Angina Pectoris   A pain in the chest related to reduced coronary circulation that may or may not involve heart or artery disease. (Greek - choking in the chest)

Anion   A negatively charged ion. An example is chloride (Cl^-)

Anoxia   No oxygen (in a tissue).

Antagonist   A drug that reacts against another. Also a muscle that has an action opposite an agonist and yields to the movement of the prime mover. (agonist).

Ante-   A prefix meaning before.

Antecubital fossa   The hollow at the front of the forearm where it meets the upper arm at the elbow, a common site for intravenous cannulation.

Anterior   Nearer to or at the front of the body. Also called ventral.

Anterior root   The structure composed of axons of motor or efferent fibres that emerges from the anterior aspect of the spinal cord and extends laterally to join a posterior root forming a spinal nerve. (Also called a ventral root).

Antibody   A substance produced by certain cells in the presence of a specific antigen that combines with that antigen to neutralise, inhibit or destroy it.

Anticoagulant   A substance that is able to delay, suppress or prevent the clotting of blood.

Antidiuretic   A substance that inhibits urine formation.

Antigen   Any substance that when introduced into the body induces the formation of antibodies or reacts with them.

Aortic body   Receptor on or near the arch of the aorta that responds to alterations in blood levels of oxygen, carbon dioxide and hydrogen ions. (A chemoreceptor).

Aortic reflex   A reflex concerned with maintaining normal general systemic blood pressure.

Apex of the heart   The caudal end of the heart.

Apnoea   Temporary or permanent cessation of breathing.

Apneuistic area   Portion of the respiratory centre in the pons that sends stimulatory impulses to the inspiratory area that activate and prolong inspiration and inhibit expiration.

Arachnoid mater   The middle of the three coverings (meninges) of the brain.

Arachnoid villus   Berry-like tuft of arachnoid mater that protrudes into the superior saggital sinus and through which the cerebrospinal fluid (CSF) enters the bloodstream.

Arrhythmia   Irregular heart rhythm. Also called a dysrhythmia.

Arteriole   A small arterial branch that delivers blood to a capillary.

Artifact   Interference or noise on an ECG tracing.

Arytenoid cartilages   A pair of small cartilages of the larynx that articulate with the cricoid cartilage.

Arteriosclerosis   A pathological condition in which the arterial walls become thickened and inelastic.

Asphyxia   Suffocation, a condition characterised by hypercarbia and hypoxaemia.

Aspirate   To remove by suction OR, to inhale a foreign body or fluid.

Association neuron   A nerve cell lying completely within the central nervous system that carries impulses from sensory neurons to motor neurons.

Astrocyte   A neuroglial cell, having a star shape, that supports neurons in the brain and spinal cord and attaches the neurons to blood vessels.

Asymptomatic   Without symptoms.

Atelectasis   A collapsed or airless state of all or part of the alveoli in the lung, which may be acute or chronic.

Atherosclerosis   A common type of arteriosclerosis affecting the coronary and cerebral arteries, characterised by the formation of plaques.

Atlas   The first cervical vertebra.

Atria   An upper chamber of the heart. (Plural - Atria). (formerly known as auricles, Latin - ear-shaped)

Atrial fibrillation   Asynchronous contraction of the atria that results in the cessation of atrial pumping.

Atropine   A parasympathetic blocking drug used to increase the heart rate in bradycardia.

Auscultation   Examination by listening to sounds in the body.

Automaticity   The spontaneous initiation of depolarising electrical impulses by pacemaker sites within the electrical conduction system of the heart.

Autonomic ganglion   A cluster of sympathetic or parasympathetic cell bodies located outside the central nervous system.

Autonomic nervous system   The subdivision of the nervous system that controls involuntary body functions. It comprises the parasympathetic and sympathetic nervous systems.

Axilla   The small hollow beneath the arm where it joins the body at the shoulder. (The armpit).

Babinski reflex   A reflex response seen in patients with brain injury. When the sole of the foot is stroked with a sharp object the big toe turns upward instead of the normal downward direction.

Bainbridge reflex   The increased heart rate that follows increased pressure or distension of the right atrium.

Baroreceptor   Nerve cell capable of responding to an increase in blood pressure. Found in the carotid sinus, the arch of the aorta and the right atrium.

Base   A compound that dissociates to form hydroxyl ions (OH⁻). A solution having a pH greater than 7.0, therefore an alkali.

Basic life support   The ABC's of CPR without adjunctive equipment.

Battle's sign   A bluish discolouration over the tip of the mastoid bone behind the ear, signifying fracture of the base of the skull.

Beta cell   A cell in the pancreatic islets (of Langerhans) that secretes insulin.

Beta receptor   A nerve centre located in the myocardium, blood vessels or bronchi that, when stimulated causes an increase in cardiac rate and contractile force, vasodilation and bronchodilation.

Bicarbonate   Any salt having two equivalents of carbonic acid to one of any base substance, usually incorrectly used as an abbreviation for sodium bicarbonate.

Bicuspid valve   The atrioventricular valve on the left side of the heart, with 2 cusps or flaps.

Bigeminy   A dysrhythmia in which every other beat is a premature contraction.

Blood-brain barrier   A mechanism that prevents the passage of unwanted materials from the blood to the cerebrospinal fluid and brain.

Blood pressure   The pressure exerted by the pulsatile flow of blood against the arterial walls. *Diastolic blood pressure* - measured during ventricular relaxation. *Systolic blood pressure* - measured during ventricular contraction.

Bolus   A single large loading dose of a drug that produces an initially higher therapeutic blood level. Also a general term for a free mass of a substance, such as food that has been swallowed.

Bradycardia   A slow heart rate, less than 60 beats per minute.

Brain stem   The portion of the brain immediately superior to the spinal cord made up of the medulla oblongata, the pons and mid-brain.

Bronchiole   A small subdivision of a bronchus.

Bronchitis   Inflammation of the bronchi characterised by hypertrophy and hyperplasia of seromucous glands and goblet cells that line the bronchi resulting in a productive cough and dyspnoea.

Bronchoconstriction   Narrowing of the bronchial tubes.

Bronchodilation   Widening of the bronchial tubes.

Bronchodilator   An agent that causes dilation of the bronchial tubes.

Bronchospasm   Severe constriction of the bronchial tree by smooth muscles.

Buffer   A substance in a fluid that tends to minimise changes in pH that would otherwise result from the addition of acid or base to the fluid.

Bundle branch block   A disturbance of the electrical conduction in the left or right bundle branch from the bundle of His.

Bundle branches   The portion of the electrical conduction system in the ventricles that conducts the depolarising impulse from the bundle of His to the Purkinje network in the myocardium. They are subdivided into the left and right bundle branches .

Bundle of His   The portion of the electrical conduction system in the interventricular septum that conducts the depolarising impulse from the atrioventricular node to the right and left bundle branches.

Calcium (Ca$^+$)   A cation required for proper functioning of heart muscle and normal bone metabolism.

Carbohydrate   An organic compound containing carbon, hydrogen and oxygen in a particular amount and arrangement and comprised of sugar subunits.)

Carbon dioxide (CO_2)   An end product of carbohydrate metabolism, eliminated from the body by respiration.

Carbon monoxide (CO)   Colourless, odourless, tasteless gas produced by incomplete combustion of organic materials.

Carboxyhaemoglobin   Haemoglobin that is combined with carbon monoxide (usually instead of oxygen).

Cardiac cycle   The events in the heart during the period from one cardiac contraction to the next.

Cardiac output   The amount of blood pumped out by the heart per minute, calculated by multiplying the stoke volume (average 70ml) by the heart rate per minute (60-80).

Cardiac reserve   The maximum percentage that cardiac output can increase above normal.

Cardiac tamponade   Embarrassment of cardiac contraction, failing cardiac output and shock caused by the accumulation of blood in the pericardium.

Cardiogenic shock   A serious complication of acute myocardial infarction in which ventricular damage is so extensive that the heart is unable to maintain adequate output to vital organs.

Cardioversion   The use of synchronised DC electric shock to convert tachyarrhythmias (eg atrial flutter) to normal sinus rhythm.

Carotid sinus   An area in the internal carotid artery, usually found just above the bifurcation of the common carotid artery, containing very sensitive nerve endings that participate in regulation of heart rate and blood pressure. Massage of this area can produce marked slowing of the heart rate, through vagal stimulation.

Carpopedal spasm   Contorted position of the hand in which the fingers flex in a claw-like attitude and the thumb curls toward the palm. A common sign of hyperventilation.

Catabolism   Chemical reactions that break down complex organic compounds into simple ones with the release of energy. (The opposite of anabolism).

Cation   A positively charged ion, eg Na^+ (sodium ion).

Cauda equina   A tail-like collection of roots of spinal nerves at the inferior end of the spinal canal.

Central neurogenic hyperventilation   An abnormal pattern of breathing seen in severe illness and injury of the brain, characterised by tachypnoea and hyperpnoea.

Cephalic   Pertaining to the head.

Cerebellum   The portion of the brain located behind and below the cerebrum, General function, co-ordination of movement.

Cerebral   Pertaining to the brain.

Cerebrum   The portion of the brain that controls higher functions such as thought, perception, memory and judgement.

Cervical   (CERVIKKAL) Pertaining to the cervix.

Cervical (CERVYCAL) Pertaining to the neck.

Chemoreceptor   Nerve cells capable of responding to a change in the concentration of chemicals such as oxygen. Found in the carotid sinus and arch of the aorta.

Cheyne-Stokes respiration   An abnormal breathing pattern characterised by rhythmic waxing and waning of the depth of respiration, with regularly occurring periods of apnoea. It is seen in association with severe central nervous system dysfunction.

CHF   An abbreviation for congestive heart failure.

Chloride   A monovalent anion important in cellular function. (Cl⁻)

Chloride shift   Diffusion of bicarbonate ions from the red blood cells to the plasma and of chloride ions from plasma into red blood cells that maintains ionic balance between red blood cells and plasma.

Cholinergic   Referring to the parasympathetic nervous system. It is derived from the word acetylcholine.

Chordae tendinae   The muscles that attach to the free edges of the three leaflets, or cusps, of the tricuspid valve and to the papillary muscles. The chordae are fibrous strands shaped like umbrella stays.

Choroid plexus   A vascular structure located in the the roof of each of the four ventricles of the brain, which produce cerebrospinal fluid.

Chronic   Applied to diseases of long duration.

Cilium   A hair-like process projecting from a cell that may be used to move the entire cell or to move substances along the surface of a cell.(Plural = cilia)

Clonic   Characterised by rapid contraction and relaxation of a muscle or group of muscles, as in grand mal epileptic fits.

Clot retraction   The consolidation of a fibrin clot, to pull damaged tissue together.

Collateral circulation   A mesh of arteries and capillaries that supply blood to a segment of tissue whose original arterial supply has been obstructed. (see infarction).

Colloid   An intravenous solution containing protein, eg Haemaccell.

Compensatory pause   The R-R interval between a premature beat and the following normal beat when this interval is longer than the R-R interval between the premature beat and the preceding normal beat. If the pause is fully compensatory, the R-R interval from the next beat together with the preceding shortened R-R interval should equal two normal R-R intervals.

Complete heart block   Third degree heart block; complete absence of conduction between the atria and the ventricles. The block can occur anywhere in the conduction system from the atrioventricular junction, AV node or bundle of His to the bundle branches. The ventricles are driven by an ectopic pacemaker below the block and atrial and ventricular contractions become dissociated.

Compliance   The ease with which the lungs and thoracic wall can be expanded.

Conductivity   The potential of the electrical conduction system of the heart to transmit electrical impulses.

Congestive heart failure   Failure of adequate ventricular function with resulting backup of blood or fluid into the lungs or body.

Constrict   To make smaller or narrower eg constricted pupils.

Constriction   Narrowing as in the term vasoconstriction the narrowing of the internal diameter of the blood vessels.

Contractility   The ability of a muscle to contract when depolarised by an electrical impulse.

Contraindication   A situation that prohibits the use of a drug, eg pregnancy or tachycardia.

Coronary   A term applied to the blood vessels of the heart that supply blood to its walls. Also loosely used to refer to an acute myocardial infarction.

Coronary sinus   A wide venous channel on the posterior surface of the heart that collects blood from the coronary circulation and returns it to the right atrium.

Corticosteroid   One of several drugs, eg prednisolone, used to counteract inflammation, whose structure is similar to that of naturally occurring steroid hormones.

Cor pulmonale   Right ventricular hypertrophy from disorders that bring about hypertension in pulmonary circulation.

Costal   Pertaining to the ribs.

Cricothyroid membrane   The membrane between the cricoid and thyroid cartilages of the larynx. The site of an emergency cricothyroidostomy.

Croup   A common disease of children, characterised by laryngeal spasm and resultant upper airway obstruction.

Crystalloid   An intravenous solution that does not contain protein, eg normal saline or Hartmanns solution.

D

Dead air space   The volume of air that that is inhaled but remains in spaces in the upper respiratory system and does not reach the alveoli to participate in gas exchange. Normally approximately 150ml. This is increased with the addition of endotracheal tubes and connectors etc.

Decussation   A crossing over: Usually refers to the crossing of most of the fibres in the large motor tracts to the opposite sides in the medullary pyramids.

Deep fascia   A sheet of connective tissue, wrapped around a muscle to hold it in place.

Dendrite   A nerve cell process carrying an impulse toward the cell body.

Depolarisation   Used in neurophysiology to describe the reduction of voltage across a cell membrane: Expressed as a movement towards less negative (more positive) voltages on the interior side of the cell membrane.

Dialysis   The process of separating crystalloids (smaller particles) from colloids (larger particles) by the difference in their rates of diffusion through a selectively permeable membrane.

Diaphoresis   Profuse perspiration.

Diaphysis   The shaft of a long bone.

Diastole   In the cardiac cycle, the phase of relaxation or dilation of the heart muscle, especially of the ventricles.

Diastolic B.P.   The force exerted by blood on arterial walls during ventricular relaxation; The lowest blood pressure measured in the large arteries approximately 80mm Hg under normal conditions for a young adult male. Usually increases in arterial disease.

Diffusion   A passive process in which there is a net or greater movement of molecules or ions from a region of high concentration to a region of low concentration until equilibrium is reached.

Dilatation   The condition or action of being dilated or expanded.

Dilate   To expand or swell.

Dissecting aneurysm   An aneurysm, or bulge, formed by the separation of the layers of the arterial wall, filled with blood.

Dissociation   Separation of inorganic acids, bases and salts into ions when dissolved in water. Also called ionisation.

Distal   Farther from the attachment of an extremity to the trunk or a structure; farther from the point of origin.

Diuretic   A chemical that increases urine volume by inhibiting reabsorption of water.

Divergence   An anatomical arrangement whereby the synaptic end-bulbs of one presynaptic neuron terminate on several post-synaptic neurons.

Dura Mater   The outer membrane (meninx) covering the brain and spinal cord.

Dyspnoea   Difficulty in breathing.

Dysrhythmia   A disturbance in cardiac rhythm.

E.C.F.   Extracellular fluid.

E.C.G.   Electrocardiogram, Electrocardiograph, Electrocardiography.

Ectopic   Located away from the normal position, such as pregnancy or focus.

Ectopic focus   A pacemaker site located in some part of the electrical conduction system other than the sino-atrial node.

Efferent neuron   A neuron that conveys impulses from the brain and spinal cord to effectors that may be either muscles or glands.

Effusion   The leakage of fluid from tissues into a cavity such as into the pleural cavity.

Electrolyte   A substance whose molecules dissociate into charged components (ions) when placed in water and is able to conduct electricity.

Embolism   A mass of solid, liquid or gaseous material that is carried in the circulation and may lead to occlusion of blood vessels with resultant infarction and necrosis of tissue supplied by those vessels.

Emphysema   Infiltration of any tissue by gas or air (surgical emphysema); a chronic pulmonary disease caused by distension of the alveoli, (due to loss of elasticity) and destructive changes in the lung parenchyma.

Endo-   A prefix meaning "inside" or "inner".

Endocardium   The thin membrane lining the inside of the heart.

Endocrine gland   A gland that secretes hormones into the blood, a ductless gland.

Endorphin   A naturally-occurring neuropeptide in the central nervous system that acts as a pain-killer.

Endothelium   The thin inner lining of blood vessels.(Also called the tunica intima)

Enzyme   A protein that acts as an organic catalyst. When myocardial tissue is damaged, enzymes from this tissue are released into the circulation. Measurement of the blood levels of these enzymes provides evidence for acute myocardial infarction.

Epigastrium   The upper middle region of the abdomen, within the sternal angle.

Epiphysis   The end of a long bone.

Epithelium   The layer of cells covering the surface of body cavities.

Erythema   Skin redness, usually caused either by engorgement of the capillaries in the lower layers of the skin or burns.

Erythrocyte   A red blood cell. The erythrocyte is the cellular element of blood that carries oxygen.

Evert   To turn a part, such as the foot or eyelid, outwards.

Excitability   The ability of the heart to initiate, conduct and be stimulated by, electrical impulses.

Exsanguinate   To bleed to death.

External respiration   The exchange of respiratory gases between the lungs and blood.

Extracellular fluid   The portion of the total body water outside the cells comprising interstitial fluid and plasma.

Extrinsic   Of external origin.

Fascia   A fibrous membrane covering supporting and separating muscles.

Febrile   Pertaining to fever or raised body temperature.

Fibrin   An insoluble protein that is essential to blood clotting; Formed from fibrinogen by the action of thrombin.

Fibrinogen   A high-molecular-weight protein in the blood that, by the action of thrombin, is converted to fibrin.

Fibrinolysis   Dissolution of a blood clot by the action of a proteolytic enzyme (such as Streptokinase) that converts insoluble fibrin into a soluble substance.

Fibrosis   The formation of fibrous tissue in place of necrotic muscle.

Fight-or-flight   The effect of stimulation of the sympathetic division of the autonomic nervous system.

Fistula   An abnormal passage between two organs or between an organ cavity and the outside.

Flaccid   Limpness of part of the body that is normally firm or rigid.

Flexor reflex   A polysynaptic reflex that withdraws a part of the body from a harmful stimulus.

Fontanelle   The openings between the bones of the skull in very young children which close as the child grows older and the bones fuse.

Foramen   A natural passage or opening; a communication between two cavities of an organ or a hole in a bone for the passage of vessels or nerves.

Fossa   A furrow or shallow depression.

Functional residual volume   The sum of residual volume and expiratory reserve volume; usually about 2,400 ml.

Ganglion   A group of nerve cell bodies that lie outside the central nervous system.

Gangrene   Local tissue death as a result of injury or cutting off the blood supply.

Gauge   A measurement of the diameter of a needle cannula. Sizes range from 12-gauge (very large) to 25-gauge (very small). The larger the gauge the smaller the lumen of the needle.

Generic name   The name given to a drug by the company that first manufactures it. Usually based on its chemical name. As opposed to its trade name.

Gland   Any organ, cell or group of cells that produces any type of secretion.

Glottis   The opening between the vocal cords.

Glucagon   A hormone produced by the pancreas that increases blood glucose level.

Glucose   A simple sugar. Its dextrose form is commonly used in intravenous infusions.

Glycogen   A highly branched polymer of glucose, containing thousands of sub-units, which functions as a compact and easily convertible store of glucose in the liver and muscle cells.

Goblet cell   A goblet-shaped unicellular gland that secretes mucus.

Heart block   A condition in which the passage of electrical impulses from the sino-atrial node through the atrioventricular node is slowed or prevented altogether. Displayed in four forms: First degree, second degree (plain and Wenckebach) and third degree.

Haematemesis   Vomiting of blood.

Haematocrit   The percentage of a sample of whole blood that is occupied by red blood cells (erythrocytes).

Haematoma   A localised collection of blood in the tissues that is a result of injury or a pierced blood vessel.

Haematuria   Blood in the urine.

Haemoglobin   The oxygen-carrying pigment of the red blood cells. When it has absorbed oxygen in the lungs, haemoglobin is bright red and is called oxyhaemoglobin. After it has given up its oxygen in the tissues it is purple and is called reduced haemoglobin.

Haemolysis   The disintegration of the red blood cells resulting from some adverse factor, such as a transfusion reaction.

Haemoptysis   Coughing up blood from the lungs.

Haemothorax   Blood in the pleural cavity.

Hemiparesis   Weakness on one side of the body.

Hemiplegia   Paralysis of one side of the body.

Hormone   A substance secreted by an endocrine gland that has effects on other organs or glands, such as insulin or testosterone.

Hygroscopic   Tending to absorb or attract water.

Hypercarbia   Excessive partial pressure of carbon dioxide in the blood.

Hyperglycaemia   Abnormally increased concentration of sugar in the blood.

Hyperkalaemia   Excessive amount of potassium in the blood.

Hyperpnoea   Increased depth of respiration.

Hyperresonance   Increased sound from percussion, as in the chest of an asthmatic.

Hypertonic   Having an osmotic pressure greater than a solution to which it is being compared, usually the intracellular fluid.

Hypertrophy   Enlargement of an organ caused by an increase in size of its constituent cells rather than an increase in the number of cells.

Hypotension   Low blood pressure.

Hypotonic   Having an osmotic pressure less than a solution to which it is being compared, usually the intracellular fluid.

Hypoxaemia   Inadequate oxygen in the blood.

Idiopathic   Of unknown cause.

Idioventricular   Relating to or affecting the ventricles only. An idioventricular rhythm arises in the ventricles

Ileum   The third portion of the small intestine.

Ilium   The broad, uppermost portion of the pelvis.

Indication   The circumstances under which a drug is suited for use.

Infant Respiratory Distress Syndrome   A disease of new-born infants, especially premature, in which insufficient amounts of surfactant are produced. Breathing is laboured due to failure of the alveoli to reinflate after collapse, due to the walls adhering to each other.

Infarction   The presence of a localised area of necrotic tissue produced by inadequate oxygenation of the tissue.

Infiltration   A deposit of fluid into the tissues, often occurring as a result of administering fluid though an IV cannula that has penetrated the opposite wall of the vein.

Inflation Reflex   Reflex that prevents over-inflation of the lungs.

Inotropic   Tending to increase the force of cardiac contractions.

Inspiratory capacity   The total inspiratory ability of the lungs. The sum of tidal volume and inspiratory reserve, about 3,600 ml

Inspiratory reserve volume   The volume of air in excess of tidal volume that can be inhaled by forced inspiration, about 3,100 ml.

Insulin   Hormone, produced by the pancreas, that reduces the blood glucose level by transporting it into the cells.

Intercalated disc   An irregular transverse thickening of sarcolemma that separates cardiac muscle fibres from each other.

Intercellular fluid   That portion of extracellular fluid that bathes the cells of the body. The internal environment of the body. Also called interstitial fluid.

Internal respiration   The exchange of respiratory gases between the blood and the cells.

Interstitial fluid   See intercellular fluid.

Intracellular   Within the cells.

Intravascular fluid   That part of the total body fluid contained within the blood vessels.

Intrinsic clotting pathway   Sequence of reactions leading to blood clotting that is initiated by the release of a substance contained within blood itself.

Inversion   The movement of the sole of the foot inward at the ankle joint.

Ion   Any charged particle or group of particles, usually formed when a substance such as a salt dissolves and dissociates.

Ischaemia   A lack of sufficient blood to a part, due to obstruction of circulation.

Islets of Langerhans   Clusters of cells in the pancreas that produce insulin.

Isotonic   Having equal tension or tone; Having equal osmotic pressure between two different solutions or between two elements in a solution.

Jaundice   The presence of excessive bile pigments in the bloodstream which give the skin, mucous membranes and eyes a distinctive yellow colour. Associated primarily with liver disease.

K⁺   The chemical symbol for potassium ion.

Ketoacidosis   The condition arising in diabetics whose insulin dose is insufficient to meet their needs wherein blood glucose reaches high levels (hyperglycaemia) and fat is metabolised to ketones and acids. It is characterised by excessive thirst, urination, nausea and vomitingsometimes coma. It may also occur in conditions other than diabetes.
Korotkoff Sounds   The sounds heard whilst taking a blood pressure.

Lactate   A salt of lactic acid.

Lactic acid   A metabolic end-product of the breakdown of glucose. It tends to accumulate when the metabolism proceeds whilst O_2 is lacking.

Laryngopharynx The inferior portion of the pharynx, extending downward from the level of the hyoid bone to divide posteriorly into the oesophagus and anteriorly into the trachea.

Lateral Farther from the midline of the body or structure.

Lesion Any abnormal local change in tissue structure or formation.

Leucocyte A white blood cell.

Leucopenia A decrease in the number of white blood cells below $5000/mm^3$

Ligament Dense, regularly arranged connective tissue that connects bones at joints.

Lignocaine A drug used to suppress ventricular ectopic activity.

Lingual frenulum A fold of mucus membrane that connects the tongue to the floor of the mouth.

Leukaemia A disease of the blood-forming organs characterised by proliferation of white blood cells and pathological changes in the bone marrow and other lymphoid tissue.

Lipid An organic compound composed of carbon, hydrogen and oxygen that is usually insoluble in water but soluble in alcohol, ether and chloroform. Examples include fats, phospholipids, steroids and prostaglandins.

Loading dose An initial large dose of a drug that provides a blood level necessary to achieve its therapeutic effects. This can then be followed my a maintenance dose.

Lumbar plexus A network formed by the anterior branches of the spinal nerves L1 to L4.

Lumen The space within a vein, artery, intestine, tube or needle.

Lymph Fluid confined in lymphatic vessels and flowing through the lymphatic system to be returned to the blood.

Lymphatic tissue A specialised form of reticular tissue that contains large numbers of lymphocytes.

Lymphocyte A type of white blood cell found in lymph nodes and tissue associated with the immune system.

Marrow Soft, sponge-like material in the cavities of bone. Red marrow produces blood cells; Yellow marrow, formed mainly of fatty tissue, has no blood producing function.

Meatus   A passage or opening, especially the external portion of a canal.

Medial   Nearer the mid-line of the body or structure.

Mediastinum   A broad median partition, actually a mass of tissue, found between the pleurae of the lungs, that extends from the sternum to the vertebral column.

Medulla   An inner layer of an organ such as the medulla of the kidneys.

Medulla oblongata   The most inferior part of the brain stem.

Medullary canal   The space within the diaphysis of a bone that contains yellow marrow.

Membrane potential   The voltage present at any instant across the cell membrane. Measured with microelectrodes inside and outside the cell, it usually registers resting values of -70mV. Also called a resting potential.

Meninges   Three membranes covering the brain and spinal cord, called the Dura Mater, Arachnoid and Pia Mater. (Singular meninx).

Metabolism   The sum of all the biochemical reactions that occur with an organism, including the synthetic (anabolic) and decomposition (catabolic) reactions.

Metaphase   The second stage of mitosis in which chromatid pairs line up on the equatorial plane of the cell.

Metastasis   The transfer of disease from one organ or part of a body to another.

Mitosis   The orderly division of the nucleus of a cell that ensures each new daughter nucleus has the same number and kind of chromosomes as the original parent nucleus. The process includes the replication of chromosomes and the distribution of t he two sets of chromosomes into two separate and equal nuclei.

Mole   The weight, in grams, of the combined atomic weights of the atoms that comprise a molecule of a substance.

Molecule   The chemical combination of two or more atoms.

Mucous membrane   A membrane that lines a body cavity that opens to the exterior. Also called the mucosa.

Mucus   The thick fluid secretion of the mucous glands and the mucous membranes. Lubricates and protects.

Murmur   An unusual heart sound; may indicate a disorder such as a malfunctioning mitral valve or may have no clinical significance.

Myelin sheath   A white, phospholipid, segmented covering formed by neurolemmocytes (Schwann cells) around the axons and dendrites of many peripheral neurons.

Myocardial infarction   Gross necrosis of myocardial tissue due to an interrupted blood supply.

Myocardium   The middle layer of the heart wall, made up of cardiac muscle, comprising the bulk of the heart and lying between the pericardium and the endocardium.

N

Na⁺   The chemical symbol for sodium ion.

NaHCO₃   The chemical symbol for sodium bicarbonate.

Naloxone   A narcotic antagonist drug used in the treatment of narcotic overdose. (Trade name Narcan).

Narcosis   An unconscious state caused by narcotics or accumulation of carbon dioxide or other toxic substances in the blood. The term usually implies respiratory depression followed by apnoea.

Nasopharynx   The superior portion of the pharynx, lying posterior to the nose and extending down to the soft palate.

Nebulisation   Treatment with medication delivered by an atomising spray.

Necrosis   Death of a cell or group of cells by disease or injury.

Negative feedback   The principle governing most control systems; a mechanism of response in which a stimulus initiates actions that reverse or reduce the stimulus.

Neonatal   Pertaining to the first four weeks after birth.

Nephron   The functional unit of the kidney.

Nerve   A cord-like bundle of nerve fibres and their associated connective tissue coursing together outside the central nervous system.

Neurogenic   Arising in or from the nervous system.

Neurogenic shock   Shock caused by massive vasodilation and pooling of blood in the peripheral vessels to the degree that adequate perfusion cannot be maintained.

Neuroglia   Cells of the nervous system that are specialised to perform the functions of connective tissue. The neuroglia of the central nervous system are the astrocytes, oligodendrocytes, microglia and ependyma; neuroglia of the peripheral nervous system include the neurolemmocytes (Schwann cells) and the ganglion satellite cells. Also called glial cells.

Neurolemma   The peripheral nucleated cytoplasmic layer of the neurolemmocyte (Schwann cell). Also called the sheath of Schwann.

Neurolemmocyte   A neuroglial cell of the peripheral nervous system that forms the myelin sheath and neurolemma of a nerve fibre by wrapping around a nerve fibre in a "swiss roll" fashion.

Neuron   A nerve cell, consisting of a cell body dendrites and an axon.

Neuropeptide   A chain of amino acids that occur naturally in the brain that acts primarily to modulate the response of or the response to a neurotransmitter. Examples are enkephalins and endorphins.

Neurotransmitter   One of a variety of molecules synthesised within the nerve axon terminals and released into the synaptic cleft in response to an action potential and affecting the membrane potential of the postsynaptic neuron.

Nicotinic receptor   Receptor found on both sympathetic and parasympathetic postganglionic neurons. So named because the actions of acetylcholine (ACh) in such receptors are similar to those produced by nicotine (stimulation).

Node of Ranvier   A space along a myelinated nerve fibre, between the individual neurolemmocytes (Schwann cells) that form the myelin sheath and the neurolemma.

Norepinephrine   A hormone secreted by the adrenal medulla that produces actions similar to those that result from sympathetic stimulation. Also called noradrenaline.

Normal saline   An intravenous solution containing 0.9% sodium chloride (NaCl) in water.

Nucleus   A spherical or ovoid organelle of a cell that contains the hereditary factors of the cell called genes: A cluster of nerve cell bodies in the central nervous system: The central portion of an atom, made up of protons and neutrons.

O2   The chemical symbol for free oxygen.

Occipital   The region of the posterior part of the head.

Occlusion   Blockage, as of a blood vessel by thrombus or clot.

Odontoid process   The tooth-like process projecting from the second cervical vertebra. (Also called the dens from the Greek - tooth)

Oligo-   A prefix from the Greek - few or deficiency.

Oligodendrocyte   A neuroglial cell that supports neurons and produces a phospholipid myelin sheath around axons of neurons of the central nervous system.

Oliguria   Minimal urine output.

Oncology   The study of tumours.

Optic chiasma   A crossing point of the optic (II cranial) nerves anterior to the pituitary gland.

Orbit   The bony, cup-shaped cavity of the skull that holds the eyeball.

Organ   A structure of definite form and function composed of two or more different kinds of tissues.

Organelle   A permanent structure within a cell with characteristic morphology that is specialised to serve a specific function in cellular activities.

Oropharynx   The second portion of the pharynx lying posterior to the mouth and extending from the soft palate down to the hyoid bone.

Orthopnoea   Dyspnoea experienced when lying down. (Usually relieved by sitting up!).

Orthostatic hypotension   Fall in blood pressure following standing up.

Osmosis   The net movement of water molecules through a selectively permeable membrane from an area of high water concentration (low solute concentration) to an area of low water concentration (high solute concentration) until equilibrium is reached.

Osmotic pressure   The pressure required to prevent the movement of pure water into a solution containing solutes when the solutions are separated by a selectively permeable membrane.

Osseous   Bony.

Otic   Pertaining to the ear

Oxidation   The removal of electrons and hydrogen ions (hydrogen atoms) from a molecule or less commonly the addition of oxygen to a molecule. The oxidation of glucose in the body is called cellular respiration.

Oxyhaemoglobin   Haemoglobin combined with oxygen.

P

Pacemaker   Specialised tissue within the heart that initiates excitation impulses.

Pacemaker site   The site in any part of the electrical conduction system of the heart where excitation impulses arise.

Palate   The horizontal structure separating the oral and nasal cavities. The roof of the mouth. (Soft palate and hard palate).

Pallor   Paleness of the skin.

Palpate   To examine by touch.

Palpitation   A sensation, felt under the left breast, of the heart skipping a beat, usually caused by premature ventricular contractions.

Palsy   Paralysis or dysfunction.

Pancreas   A soft oblong organ lying along the greater curvature of the stomach and connected by, usually, two ducts to the duodenum. It is both exocrine (secreting pancreatic juice) and endocrine (secreting insulin, glucagon and somatostatin).

Papillary muscle   Protrusions of the myocardium into the ventricular cavities to which the chordae tendinae are attached.

Para-   Prefix meaning beside or part(ly).

Paradoxical breathing   The situation in which attempts to inhale cause collapse of a portion of the chest wall instead of expansion. It is seen in flail chest.

Paraplegia   Paralysis of the lower half of the body.

Parasthaesia   An abnormal sensation, often of the pins and needles variety, indicating disturbance in nerve function.

Parasympathetic division   One of the two subdivisions of the autonomic nervous system, having cell bodies of preganglionic neurons in nuclei in the brain stem and the lateral grey matter of the sacral portion of the spinal cord. Primarily concerned with activities that restore and conserve body energy and involuntary vegetative functions. Mediated largely by the vagus nerve through the chemical acetylcholine.

Parathyroid gland   One of four small endocrine glands embedded on the posterior surfaces of the lateral lobes of the thyroid gland.

Parathyroid hormone   A hormone secreted by the parathyroid glands that decreases blood phosphate level and increases blood calcium level.

Parenchyma   The functional parts of any organ, as opposed to tissue that forms its ground substance or framework.

Parenteral   Situated or occurring outside the intestines, referring to introduction of substances into the body other than by way of the intestines such as intradermal, subcutaneous, intramuscular, intravenous or intraspinal.

Parietal   Pertaining to or forming the outer wall of a body cavity.

Parietal lobe   The portion of the brain containing sensory areas and areas of muscle control.

Parietal pleura   The outer layer of the serous pleural membrane that encloses and protects the lungs. The layer that is attached to the wall of the pleural cavity.

Paroxysm   A sudden periodic attack or recurrence of symptoms of a disease.

Patent   Open, unobstructed.

Pathogenesis   The development of a disease or a morbid or pathological state.

Pathogen   A disease-producing organism.

PCO2   The symbol for the partial pressure of carbon dioxide in a gaseous mixture.

PEEP   Positive end-expiratory pressure. As in ventilation of a patient.

Pelvic cavity   Inferior portion of the abdominopelvic cavity that contains the urinary bladder, sigmoid colon, rectum and internal female and male reproductive structures.

Percussion   Striking a part of a patients body with short, sharp blows in order to produce a sound that will indicate the condition of the structures within.

Percutaneous   Through the skin.

Perfusion   The flow of blood or liquid through tissues.

Pericardial cavity   Small potential space between the visceral and parietal layers of the serous pericardium.

Pericardial effusion   Excess fluid within the pericardial sac.

Pericardial tamponade   An accumulation of excess fluid or blood in the pericardial sac that interferes with heart action. Causes electro-mechanical dissociation. Also known as cardiac tamponade.

Pericardium   A loose-fitting membrane that encloses the heart, consisting of an outer fibrous layer and an inner serous layer.

Periosteum   The membrane that covers bone and is essential for bone growth, repair and nutrition.

Peripheral   Pertaining to an outer surface.

Peripheral nervous system   That part of the nervous system that lies outside the central nervous system - nerves and ganglia.

Peripheral resistance   The hindrance to blood flow due to friction between blood and blood vessels, related to viscosity of blood and diameter, roughness and length of blood vessels.

Peritoneum   The largest serous membrane of the body, that lines the abdominal cavity and covers the viscera.

Peritonitis   inflammation of the peritoneum.

pH   A symbol of the measure of the concentration of hydrogen ions in a solution. The pH scale extends from 0 to 14, with a value of 7 expressing neutrality, values lower than 7 expressing increased acidity and values higher than 7 expressing increased alkalinity.

Pharynx   The throat; a tube that starts at the internal nares and runs partway down the neck where it opens into the oesophagus posteriorly and into the larynx anteriorly.

Phaechromocytoma   Tumour of the chromaffin cells of the adrenal medulla that results in hypersecretion of medullary hormones. A contraindication to glucagon in drug form.

Phlebitis   Inflammation of the wall of a vein, sometimes caused by the presence of an IV line, characterised by tenderness, redness and slight oedema along the line of the vein.

Pia mater   The inner membrane (meninx) covering the brain and spinal cord.

Pituitary gland   A small endocrine gland lying in the sella turcica of the sphenoid bone and attached to the hypothalamus by the infundibulum. It influences the secretions of all the other glands in the body.

Plasma   The extracellular fluid found in the blood vessels. Blood minus the formed elements.

Plasma membrane   Outer limiting membrane that separates the cells internal parts from extracellular fluid and the external environment.

Pleura   The serous membrane that enfolds the lungs and lines the walls of the chest and diaphragm.

Pleural cavity   Small potential space between the visceral and parietal pleurae.

Plexus   A network of nerves, veins or lymphatic vessels.

Pneumotaxic area   Portion of the respiratory centre in the pons that continually sends inhibitory impulses to the inspiratory area to limit inspiration and facilitate expiration.

PO2   The symbol for the partial pressure of oxygen in a gaseous mixture.

Polarised   A condition in which opposite effects or states exist at the same time. In electrical contexts having one portion positive and one negative. For example a polarised nerve cell membrane has the outer surface positively charged and the inner surface negatively charged.

Pons   The portion of the brain stem that forms a bridge between the medulla and the midbrain anterior to the cerebellum.

Posterior   Nearer to or at the back of the body. Also called dorsal.

Postganglionic neuron   The second visceral efferent neuron in an autonomic pathway, having its cell body and dendrites located in an autonomic ganglion and its unmyelinated axon ending at cardiac muscle, smooth muscle or a gland.

Postictal   Referring to the period after a fit.

Postsynaptic neuron   The nerve cell that is activated by a neurotransmitter substance from another neuron and carries action potentials away from the synapse.

Potentiation   Enhancement of the effects of one drug by another.

Pre-eclampsia   A syndrome characterised by sudden hypertension, large amounts of protein in urine and generalised oedema. It might be related to an autoimmune or allergic reaction due to the presence of a foetus.

Preganglionic neuron   The first visceral efferent neuron in an autonomic pathway with its cell body and dendrites in the brain or spinal cord and its myelinated axon ending at an autonomic ganglion where it synapses with a postganglionic neuron.

Premature   Descriptive of a baby born before the eighth month of pregnancy or less than 2kg (51/2 lb)

Presynaptic neuron   A nerve cell that carries an action potential towards a synapse.

P-R interval   The period of time between the start of the P wave and the start of the QRS complex. Normally 0.12 to 0.20 of a second.

Prolapse   A dropping, falling down or turning out of an organ especially the uterus or rectum.

Pronation   A movement of the flexed forearm in which the palm of the hand is turned posteriorly.

Prophase   The first stage in mitosis in which chromatid pairs are formed and aggregate around the equatorial plane region of the cell.

Prophylaxis   Measures taken to prevent the occurrence of a disease or abnormal state.

Proprioception   The receipt of information from muscles, tendons and the labyrinth that enables the brain to determine movements and position of the body and parts. Also called kinesthesia.

Protein   An organic compound consisting of carbon, hydrogen, oxygen, nitrogen and sometimes sulphur and phosphorus and made up of amino acids linked by peptide bonds.

Prothrombin   An inactive protein synthesised by the liver, released into the blood and converted to active thrombin in the process of blood clotting.

Proximal   Nearer the attachment of an extremity to the body or a structure; nearer the point of origin.

Pulmonary   Concerning or affected by the lungs.

Pulmonary oedema   An abnormal accumulation of interstitial fluid in the tissue spaces and alveoli of the lungs due to an increased pulmonary capillary permeability or increased pulmonary capillary pressure.

Pulmonary embolism   The presence of a blood clot or other foreign substance in a pulmonary arterial blood vessel that obstructs circulation to lung tissue.

Pulse pressure   The difference between the maximum (systolic) and minimum (diastolic) blood pressures. Normally a value of about 40mm Hg.

P wave   The deflection wave of an electrocardiogram that records atrial depolarisation.

Pyrexia   A condition in which the body temperature is above normal.

QRS complex   Deflection of the ECG caused by ventricular depolarisation.

Quadrant   One of four parts.

Quadriplegia   Paralysis of both arms and both legs.

Q wave   The first downward deflection (negative) of the QRS complex not preceded by an R wave.

Radial   Pertaining to the wrist or arranged as the spokes of a wheel.

Rales   Abnormal breath sounds produced by flow of air through constricted, oedematous or fluid-filled small airways.

Reactivity   The ability of an antigen to react specifically with the antibody whose formation it induced.

Receptor   A specialised cell or nerve cell terminal modified to respond to some specific sensory stimulus, such as touch, cold, light, pressure or sound. A specific molecule or arrangement of molecules organised to accept only molecules with a complementary structure.

Reciprocal innervation   The phenomenon whereby impulses stimulate contraction of one muscle and simultaneously inhibit contraction of antagonistic muscles.

Rectum   The last 20cm (8") of the gastrointestinal tract, from the sigmoid colon to the anus.

Referred pain   The pain apparently felt at a site remote from the site of origin, such as pain in the arm originating from angina or the pain in the hip from a knee injury.

Reflex   Fast response to a change in the internal or external environment that attempts to restore homeostasis. It passes over a reflex arc.

Reflex arc   The most basic conduction pathway through the nervous system, connecting a receptor and an effector and consisting of a receptor, a sensory neuron, a centre in the central nervous system for a synapse, a motor neuron and an effector.

Refractory period   (Absolute) A time during which an excitable cell cannot respond to a stimulus that is usually adequate to provoke an action potential, even a stronger than normal stimulus. (Relative) The stage of ventricular diastole during which the cardiac muscle is repolarising to a resting state following depolarisation. During this period of the refractory period the heart can be stimulated to contract prematurely.

Regurgitation   The emptying of the stomach contents through the mouth, without the muscular effort of vomiting.

Renal   Pertaining to the kidney.

Repolarisation   The electrical process of recharging depolarised muscle fibres back to the resting state.

Residual volume   The volume of air still contained in the lungs after a maximal expiration; about 1200ml

Resistance   The ability to ward off disease: The hindrance encountered by an electrical charge as it passes through a substance from one point to another: The hindrance encountered by blood as it flows through the vascular system or by air through respiratory passages.

Respiration   Overall exchange of gases between the atmosphere, blood and body cells, consisting of pulmonary ventilation, external respiration and internal respiration.

Respiratory centre   Neurons in the reticular formation of the brain stem that regulate the rate of respiration.

Respiratory distress syndrome of the newborn   A disease of newborn infants, especially in prematurity, in which insufficient amounts of surfactant are produced and breathing is laboured due to unrelieved alveolar collapse.

Resting potential   The voltage that exists between the inside and outside of a cell membrane when the cell is not responding to a stimulus. (About -70 mV) with the inside of the cell negative.

Reticular formation   A network of small groups of nerve cells scattered among bundles of fibres, beginning in the medulla as a continuation of the spinal cord and extending upwards through the central part of the brain stem.

Reticulocyte   An immature red blood cell.

Rh factor   An inherited agglutinogen on the surface of red blood cells.

Rhinology   The study of the nose and its disorders.

Rhonchi   Coarse rattling sounds heard in the chest, caused by excessive secretions in the bronchi.

Right heart failure   An inability of the right ventricle to pump blood forward effectively, causing a back-up of blood in the systemic veins, with consequent oedema of body tissues.

Right heart (atrial) reflex   A reflex concerned with maintaining normal venous blood pressure.

Rigor mortis   State of partial contraction of muscles following death due to lack of ATP (adenosine triphosphate) that causes cross bridges of thick myofilaments to remain attached to thin myofilaments, thus preventing relaxation.

R on T   A dangerous type of premature ventricular contraction, that is seen on the ECG to fall on the T wave of the previous QRS-T complex, representing the occurrence of an extrasystole during the vulnerable period of ventricular repolarisation and often triggering ventricular tachycardia or ventricular fibrillation.

Rugae   Large folds in the mucosa of an empty hollow organ such as the stomach and vagina.

R wave   The positive deflection in the QRS complex.

R$_x$ An abbreviation meaning prescription or "I prescribe".

S

Saddle joint   A synovial joint in which the articular surfaces of both the bones are saddle shaped or concave in one direction and convex in the other direction, as in the joint between the trapezium and the metacarpal in the thumb.

Saliva   A clear, alkaline, somewhat viscous secretion produced by the three pairs of salivary glands. Takes part in digestion.

Salicylate   The class of drugs that includes aspirin.

Saline   A solution containing Sodium Chloride (NaCl). Normal saline contains 0.9% NaCl, the same proportion as normal body fluids.

Saltatory conduction   The propagation of an action potential (nerve impulse) along the exposed portions of a myelinated nerve fibre. The action potential appears at successive neurofibral nodes (Nodes of Ranvier) and therefore seems to jump from n ode to node.

SA node   An abbreviation for sino-atrial node.

Sarcolemma   The cell membrane of a muscle cell especially of a skeletal muscle cell.

Sarcomere   A contractile unit in a striated muscle cell extending from one Z line to the next Z line.

Sarcoplasm   The cytoplasm of a muscle cell.

Saturated fat   A fat that contains no double bonds between any of its carbon atoms. All are single bonds and all carbon atoms are bonded to the maximum number of hydrogen atoms. Found naturally in animal foods such as meat, milk, milk products and eggs.

Schwann cell   A neuroglial cell of the peripheral nervous system that forms the myelin sheath and neurolemma of a nerve fibre by wrapping around a nerve fibre in a swiss roll fashion.

Sclera   The tough white covering of the eyeball.

Sclerosis   A hardening with loss of elasticity, of tissue.

Scoliosis   An abnormal lateral curvature from the normal vertical line of the spine. Causes a "hunchback".

Selectively permeable membrane   A membrane that permits the passage of certain substances, but restricts the passage of others.

Sella turcica   A depression on the superior surface of the sphenoid bone that houses the pituitary gland.

Semilunar valve   A valve guarding the entrance into the aorta or the pulmonary trunk from a ventricle of the heart. Called semi-lunar as it has two half-moon shaped flaps.

Sensory area   A region of the cerebral cortex concerned with the interpretation of sensory impulses.

Septum   A wall dividing two cavities, as is the heart and nose.

Serous membrane   A membrane that lines body cavities, that does not open to the exterior and is lubricated with serous fluid. Found in the pleural, pericardial and peritoneal cavities.

Serum   Plasma minus its clotting proteins, found after clot formation.

Sesamoid bones   Small seed-shaped bones, usually found in tendons, such as the patella.

Shock   A state of inadequate tissue perfusion which may be caused by pump failure (cardiogenic shock), volume loss (hypovolaemic shock), vasodilation (neurogenic shock), allergic reaction (anaphylactic shock), or any combination of these.

Shunt   A situation when the blood returns to the heart from the lungs without being oxygenated caused by, among other things, atelectasis or pulmonary oedema.

Silent M.I.   Painless myocardial infarction occurring in 10 - 20% of patients with M.I. especially the elderly.

Sinoatrial node   A compact mass of cardiac muscle cells specialised for conduction located in the right atrium beneath the opening of the superior vena cava. The normal pacemaker of the heart.

Sinus   A hollow in a bone or other tissue, a channel for blood, any cavity having a narrow opening.

Sinus bradycardia   Sinus rhythm with a rate of less than 60 beats per minute.

Sinus tachycardia   Sinus rhythm with a rate of more than 100 beats per minute.

Sliding filament theory   The most commonly accepted explanation for muscle contraction, in which actin and myosin myofilaments move into interdigitation with each other, decreasing the length of the sarcomere and therefore contracting the muscle.

Sodium   The main cation (+ion) of the extracellular fluid. Chemical symbol Na^+.

Sodium bicarbonate   ($NaHCO_3$), A chemical buffer used to increase pH when acidosis is present.

Sodium-potassium pump   An active transport system located in the cell membrane that transports sodium ions out of the cell and potassium ions into the cell at a cost of cellular ATP. It functions to keep the ionic concentrations at physiological levels.

Solution   A homogenous molecular or ionic dispersion of one or more substances (solutes) in a usually liquid dissolving medium (solvent).

Somatic nervous system   The portion of the peripheral nervous system made up of the somatic (voluntary) efferent fibres that run between the central nervous system and the skeletal muscles.

Spasm   An involuntary convulsive muscular contraction.

Sphincter   A circular muscle constricting an orifice.

Spleen   A large mass of lymphatic tissue between the fundus of the stomach and the diaphragm that functions in phagocytosis, production of lymphocytes, blood storage and destruction of old red blood cells.

Spontaneous pneumothorax   A rupture of the lung parenchyma, without trauma, leading to air in the pleural cavity. Prevalent among tall, thin, dark, young men.

Starlings law   The force of muscular contraction is determined by the length of the stretched cardiac muscle fibres; the greater the length of the stretched fibres, the greater the force of the contraction.

Stat.   A abbreviation meaning immediately.

Status asthmaticus   A severe, prolonged asthmatic attack that cannot easily be broken.

Status epilepticus   The occurrence of two or more epileptic fits without a period of full consciousness between.

Stenosis   An abnormal narrowing or constriction of a duct or opening.

Stimulus   A change in the environment that is capable of altering a membrane potential.

Stoma   A small opening, especially an artificially created opening, such as that made by tracheostomy, ileostomy or colostomy.

Stretch receptor   Receptor, e.g. in the walls of bronchi, bronchioles and lungs that sends impulses to the respiratory centre, that prevents overinflation of the lungs.

Stricture   Narrowing of a duct or natural passage by inflammation.

Stridor   A harsh, high-pitched respiratory sound associated with severe upper airway obstruction, such as laryngeal oedema.

Stroke volume   The volume of blood expelled by the ventricles in one beat; about 70ml.

S - T segment   The interval between the QRS complex and the beginning of the T wave. It is often elevated or depressed in severe myocardial ischaemia.

Subarachnoid space   A space, between the arachnoid and pia mater that surrounds the brain and spinal cord, through which cerebro-spinal fluid circulates.

Subcutaneous   Beneath the skin. Also known as sub-cut or SQ.

Subcutaneous emphysema   A condition in which trauma to the lung or airway results in the escape of air into tissues of the body, especially the chest wall, neck or face, causing a crackling sensation on palpation of the skin.

Subdural space   A space, between the dura mater and the arachnoid of the brain and spinal cord, that contains a small amount of fluid.

Subthreshold stimulus   A stimulus of weak intensity that cannot initiate an action potential. Also called a subliminal stimulus.

Sulcus   A groove or depression between parts, especially between the convolutions of the brain.

Supinate   To turn the forearm so that the palm faces upward.

Supine   Lying flat on one's back, face upward.

Suppuration   Pus formation and discharge.

Supraventricular tachycardia   Tachycardia arising from a pacemaker site above the ventricles.

Surfactant   A phospholipid substance produced by the septal cells in the alveoli that reduces surface tension and therefore prevents atelectasis.

Suture   A fibrous joint, especially in the skull, where bone surfaces are closely united. Also a wound closure after surgery

S wave   The first downward deflection of the QRS complex that is preceded by an R wave.

Sympathetic division   One of the two divisions of the autonomic nervous system, having cell bodies of preganglionic neurons in the lateral grey columns of the thoracic segment and first two or three lumbar segments of the spinal cord. Primarily concerned with processes involving the expenditure of energy.

Sympathomimetic   Producing effects that mimic the effects of the sympathetic division of the autonomic nervous system.

Symphysis   A line of union. A slightly moveable cartilaginous joint such as the symphysis pubis between the anterior surfaces of the pubic bones.

Synapse   The junction between the process of two adjacent neurons. The place where the activity of one neuron affects the activity of the other.

Synaptic cleft   The narrow gap that separates the axon terminal of one nerve cell from another nerve cell or muscle fibre (cell) and across which a neurotransmitter diffuses to affect the postsynaptic cell.

Synaptic delay   The length of time between the arrival of the action potential at the axon terminal and the membrane potential change on the postsynaptic membrane; usually about 0.5 ms.

Synaptic end-bulb   Expanded distal end of an axon terminal that contains synaptic vesicles.

Synaptic vesicle   Membrane-enclosed sac in a synaptic end-bulb that stores neurotransmitter substances.

Syncope   A temporary loss of consciousness, commonly due to cerebral ischaemia or postural hypotension. A faint.

Syndrome   A group of signs and symptoms that occur together in a pattern characteristic of a particular disease.

Syneresis   The process of clot retraction.

Synergism   The combined effect of two or more drugs such that their action in combination is greater than the sum of their individual actions.

Synovial cavity   The space between the articulating bones of a synovial or diarthrotic joint, filled with synovial fluid.

System   An association of organs that have a common function.

Systemic   Affecting the whole body; generalised.

Systemic circulation   The routes through which oxygenated blood flows from the left ventricle through the aorta to all the organs of the body and deoxygenated bloods returns to the right atrium.

Systole   In the cardiac cycle, the phase of contraction of the heart muscle, especially of the ventricles.

Tachypnoea   An excessively rapid rate of breathing.

Tendon   A white, fibrous cord of dense, regularly arranged connective tissue that attaches muscle to bone.

Tension pneumothorax   The situation in which air enters the pleural space through a one- way valve defect in the lung, causing progressive increase in intrapleural pressure, lung collapse and impairment of circulation.

Tetanus   An infectious disease caused by the toxin of Clostridium Tetani, characterised by tonic muscle spasms and exaggerated reflexes, lockjaw and arching of the back. Also a smooth sustained contraction produced by a series of very rapid stimuli to a muscle.

Tetany   A nervous condition caused by hypoparathyroidism and subsequent hypercalcaemia, characterised by intermittent or continuous tonic muscular contractions of the extremities.

Thoracolumbar outflow   The fibres of the sympathetic preganglionic neurons which have their cell bodies in the lateral grey columns of the thoracic segments and first two or three lumbar segments of the spinal cord.

Threshold potential   The membrane voltage that must be reached in order to trigger an action potential (nerve impulse)

Threshold stimulus   Any stimulus strong enough to initiate an action potential (nerve stimulus).

Thrombin   The active enzyme, formed from prothrombin, that acts to convert fibrinogen to fibrin.

Thrombocyte   A fragment of cytoplasm enclosed in a cell membrane and lacking a nucleus, found in the circulating blood. Plays a role in blood clotting. Also called a platelet.

Thromboplastin   A factor or collection of factors whose action initiates the blood clotting process.

Thrombosis   The abnormal formation of a clot, (thrombus) in an unbroken blood vessel.

Thrombus   A clot formed in an unbroken blood vessel.

Thyroid cartilage   The largest single cartilage of the larynx, consisting of two fused plates that form the anterior wall of the larynx. Also called the Adam's apple.

Thyroid gland   An endocrine gland with right and left lateral lobes on either side of the trachea, connected by an isthmus located in front of the trachea just below the cricoid cartilage.

TIA   An abbreviation for transient ischaemic attack.

Tidal volume   The volume of air moved in and out in any one breath; about 500ml in quiet breathing at rest.

Tissue   A group of cells and their intercellular substance joined together to perform a specific function.

Tonsil   A multiple aggregation of large lymphatic nodules embedded in the mucous membrane of the pharynx.

Total body water (TBW)   The total fluid content of the body; about 60% of body weight in adult males.

Total lung capacity   The sum of tidal volume, expiratory reserve volume and residual volume; About 6000 ml. in an adult male.

Toxic   Pertaining to poison; Poisonous.

Toxoid   A chemically modified toxin that, when injected, stimulates the development of immunity against a specific disease but that is not in itself harmful. e.g. tetanus toxoid.

Trachea   Tubular air passageway extending from the larynx to the fifth thoracic vertebra.

Transverse fissure   The deep cleft that separates the cerebrum from the cerebellum.

Trendelenburg position   The position in which a patient is placed, on his back, with legs raised and head lowered.

Tricuspid valve The atrioventricular valve on the right side of the heart. So-called as it has three flaps or cusps.

Tropic hormone A hormone whose target is another endocrine gland.

Tunica adventitia The outer coat of an artery or vein, composed mainly of elastic and collagenous fibres.

Tunica intima The inner coat of an artery or vein, consisting of a smooth lining of endothelium and its supporting layer of connective tissue.

Tunica media The middle layer of an artery or vein, composed of smooth muscle and elastic fibres.

T wave The deflection of an ECG that records ventricular repolarisation.

U

Ulcer An open lesion of the skin or mucous membrane, with loss of substance and necrosis of the tissue.

Unifocal Arising from a single site.

Unsaturated fat A fat that contains one or more covalent bonds between its carbon atoms. E.g. peanut oil, corn oil, olive oil.

Uraemia Accumulation of toxic levels of urea and other nitrogenous waste products in the blood, usually resulting from severe kidney malfunction.

Ureter One of the two tubes that connect the kidneys to the bladder.

Urethra The duct from the bladder to the outside of the body.

Uvula A soft, fleshy mass especially the V-shaped pendant part descending from the soft palate.

V

Vagal activity Parasympathetic activity.

Valvular stenosis A narrowing of a heart valve, especially the mitral valve.

Varicose Pertaining to an unnatural swelling and hardening, particularly of the superficial lower leg veins.

Vasoconstriction A decrease in the size of the lumen of a blood vessel

Vasodilation An increase in the size of the lumen of a blood vessel.

Vasomotor centre A cluster of neurons in the medulla that controls the diameter of blood vessels, particularly arteries.

Vein A blood vessel that carries blood back to the heart.

Venule A small vein that collects blood from the capillaries and delivers it to a vein.

Villus A projection of the intestinal mucous cells containing connective tissue, blood vessels and a lymphatic vessel. It functions in the absorption of food. Also found in the chorion part of the placenta, there known as the chorionic villi. Also found in the subarachnoid space, as a projection of the arachnoid mater, there known as an arachnoid villus.

Viscera The organs inside the ventral body cavity.

Visceral The surface of an organ or structure that is nearer the inside of the body.

Vital capacity The sum of inspiratory reserve volume, tidal volume and expiratory reserve volume; On average about 4,800 ml.

Vocal folds A pair of mucous membrane folds in the larynx, below the ventricular folds, that function in voice production.

W

Wandering macrophage Phagocytic cell that develops from a monocyte, leaves the blood and then migrates to infected tissue.

White matter Aggregations or bundles of myelinated axons located in the brain and spinal cord.

X

Xiphoid process The lowest part of the sternum.

Z

Zygoma The cheek bone.